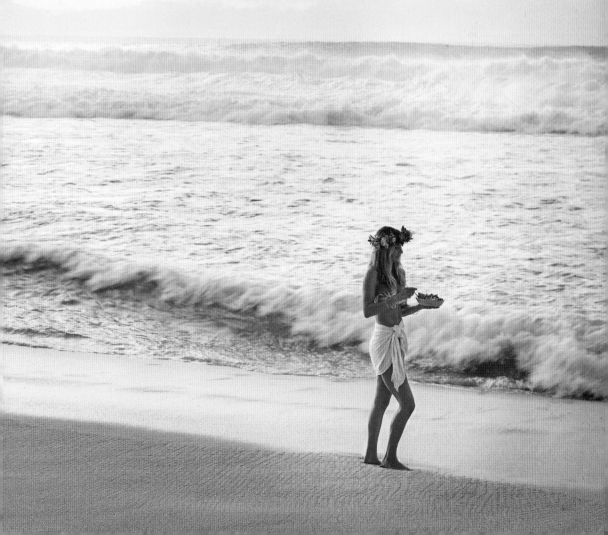

plant
over processed

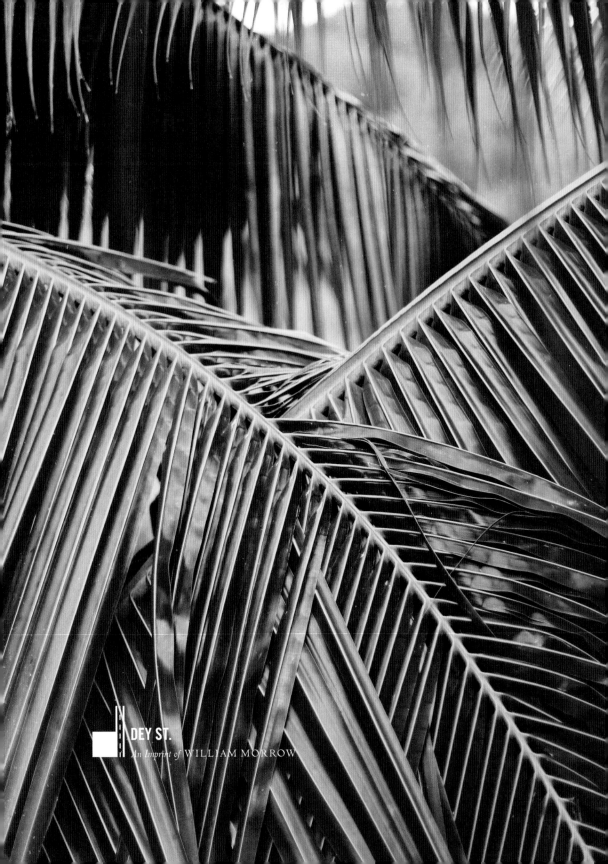

DEY ST.
An Imprint of WILLIAM MORROW

plant
over processed

75 SIMPLE & DELICIOUS PLANT-BASED RECIPES
FOR NOURISHING YOUR BODY AND EATING FROM THE EARTH

Andrea
Hannemann

PHOTOGRAPHY BY PETRINA TINSLAY

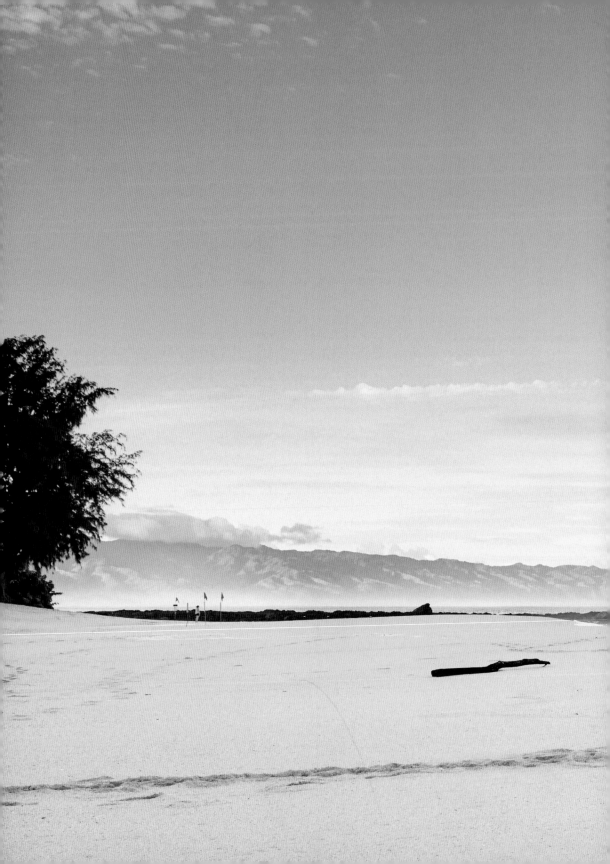

To all those out there in search of friendly support, healthy inspiration, and deliciously nutritious recipes: This book is for you!

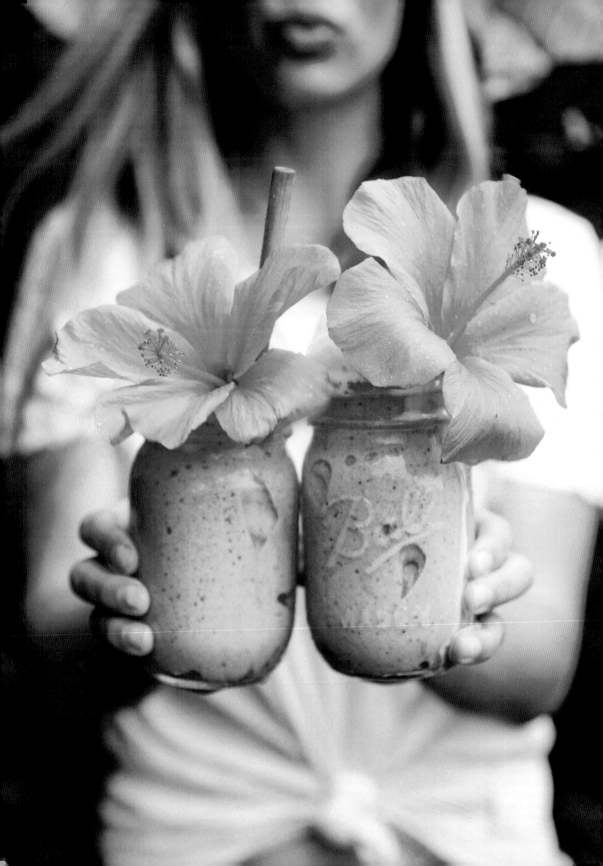

contents

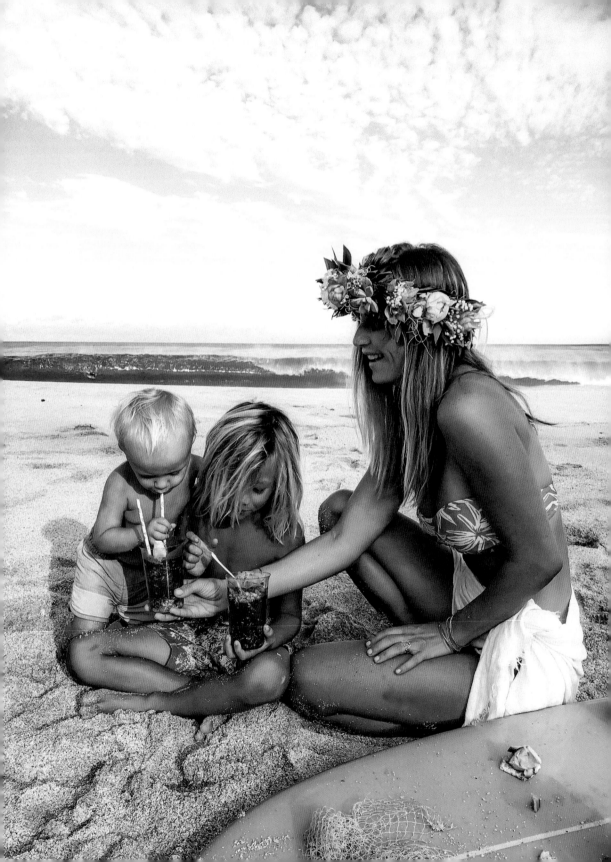

introduction
my plant-based path—and yours!

Aloha, I'm Andy! I was born in Saskatchewan, Canada, but my heart has always belonged to the tropics. Growing up, I dreamed of living near the ocean, learning to surf, and spending time on the beach. In high school, I wore a puka shell necklace, painted waves on my bedroom walls, and even decorated my room with a fake palm tree and a picture of surfer Kelly Slater. I had only seen Hawaii in the movies and in magazines—until the day my dad announced that the family was taking a trip there!

I'll never forget landing in Honolulu and stepping off the plane. The air was warm and thick with the scent of plumerias—a stark contrast to scraping ice off the windshield of my parents' car and walking in knee-deep snow the morning before! I remember begging my dad to let me go to the beach on the night we arrived, and as I walked toward the water, I was in heaven. This was the first time I'd heard the sound of the ocean or felt sand under my feet. I was hooked! After that family vacation, I knew I had to get back to

Hawaii, and eventually I did. At eighteen, after applying to college in Hawaii twice, I was finally accepted, and I packed my bags and moved to the North Shore of Oahu.

I moved for the beach and the weather, but little did I know that I'd meet a surfer boy who would become my partner in love and life! Shem and I got engaged a week after we first locked eyes and we married shortly afterward. Fast-forward fourteen years, and today we are living on the North Shore with our three rambunctious boys: Tama, eleven, Ira, seven, and Nalu, one.

Our life is wild and simple—and I mean simple. We live in a small house across the street from the beach with an outdoor shower. Our town has one main road, with mountains on one side and the beach on the other, and roosters are our alarm clock. We spend our free time surfing, skateboarding (the boys, not me), traveling, and enjoying meals as a family and with friends. I'm sure you've heard the typical Hawaiian sayings "Live with Aloha" and "Hang Loose." These are the mantras of the Hawaiian Islands and the concepts we live by. I'd translate them, roughly, as "Live your life guided by love and those you love" and "Don't forget to smell the flowers along the way."

My health, on the other hand, wasn't always so simple. Starting in my teens, I struggled with a long list of health issues, including irritable bowel syndrome, celiac disease, irregular menstrual cycles, hypothyroidism, asthma, and skin problems. For years I spent money on specialists and experimented with various diets, supplements, and medications in hopes of alleviating my issues. Occasionally something I tried would help, but never for long, and my cycle of health problems would always return. Most days I would wake up and go to bed with a stomachache. My digestive issues were such a problem that I avoided eating during the day and only ate once I got home at night, knowing that at least I could lie down and be close to a toilet (I know, TMI!). My hormones and reproductive system were also completely out of whack. At one point I was having a full menstrual cycle every other week for seven months straight. It became impossible to lead a normal life. I put on a happy face, exercised every day, and did what I could to be an involved mother and wife. But inside I was struggling, counting down the hours just to get through the day. It was no way to live.

In January of 2015, I decided I had to make a change. One night, as I was lying awake contemplating my health issues, I had a moment of clarity: No doctor or specialist was going to solve this for me. I needed to take things into my own hands, and it was up to me to research my health issues. I would use professionals as resources, but I needed to listen to my intuition and what my body was telling me. I had discovered a number of people online who were following plant-based diets and had experienced full health transformations as a result. I had also been reading that fruits and vegetables were the gentlest foods for a sensitive digestive system. However, the idea of following a strict vegan diet seemed outlandish. I had convinced myself that eating fruits, vegetables, and starches caused me to bloat, so I avoided these foods like the plague, instead consuming what was advertised as "healthy"—animal protein, protein bars, and health drinks loaded with artificial sweeteners—while also attempting to satisfy my unruly sweet tooth with candy bars. I wouldn't allow myself even a bite of a banana or a blueberry, for fear of how my digestive system would react. I thought that I was making relatively healthy choices and doing what was best for my body.

In spite of my fears, I decided to give a plant-based diet a try for thirty days. Eating 100 percent plant-based, where many of my calories would come from vegetables, fruits, and starches, seemed to fly in the face of everything I'd been taught. At the same time,

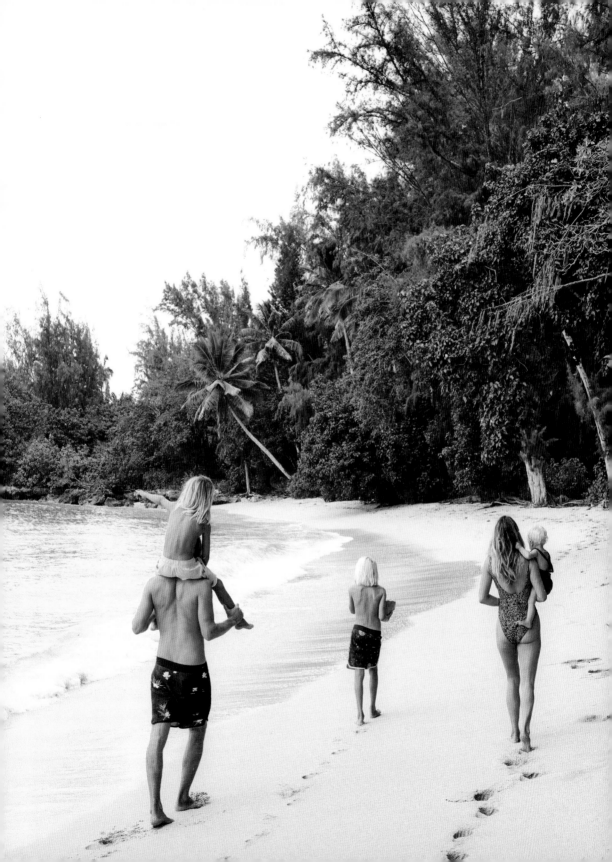

a little voice inside of me was asking, "Why would these fruits and vegetables and grains come from the earth if they weren't meant to benefit us?" It was as if my heart was telling my brain, "Just stop thinking and start trusting!" I also decided to eliminate all processed foods from my diet during this thirty-day period, eating only foods that came from the earth.

I will give more detail on exactly what I ate—and what you should eat if you want to do what I did—in the next chapters. But in a nutshell, I made it my daily goal to eat more plants than processed foods. This is where my mantra, "Plant Over Processed," was born. Specifically, I was aiming to get 80 percent of my daily calories from living plant foods, and I would use what I had learned about food combining (more on this concept later) to get the most out of these foods and my efforts. To accomplish this, I decided to eat the first two meals of my day predominantly or completely raw: breakfast was a digestion-boosting tonic followed by a nourishing green smoothie; and lunch was a big green salad with fruits, veggies, and nuts and/or another smoothie. Dinner was a cooked plant-based meal—perhaps a soup or curry, a vegan stir-fry, or a roasted veggie burrito. Snacks were also 100 percent plant-based. The idea was to eat as gently and as naturally as possible, in hopes that my body could accept these foods and heal. I figured that if it takes the body approximately thirty minutes to digest a serving of fruits and

vegetables, versus eighteen to twenty-four hours to digest meat, my body could use that extra energy to heal. My goal was to feel normal. I never imagined that I would feel like an entirely new, healthy, energized person at the end of this thirty-day trial!

The first big change I noticed was with my digestion. I went from feeling bloated pretty much all the time to feeling good for the first time ever! I would go on to learn that health starts in your gut. When your gut is happy, everything else benefits, resulting in clearer skin, decreased inflammation, more energy, better mental clarity, and improved mood, not to mention a flatter stomach and an overall more toned physique. I felt like I was unlocking the real me that had been hidden away for all those years!

I initially kept my thirty-day experiment a secret, thinking that if no one noticed the new way I was eating, it was a good sign. It would mean that eating 100 percent plant-based was compatible with other aspects of my life. I come from a long line of carnivores, and my husband's family owns a chain of burger restaurants, which Shem was managing at the time! So you can imagine how extreme a plant-based diet would have sounded to those around me. To my surprise, keeping it a secret was actually quite easy, and that taught me something: No one really cares what you're eating! So make it work for you. I have plenty of tips on how to pull off sticking

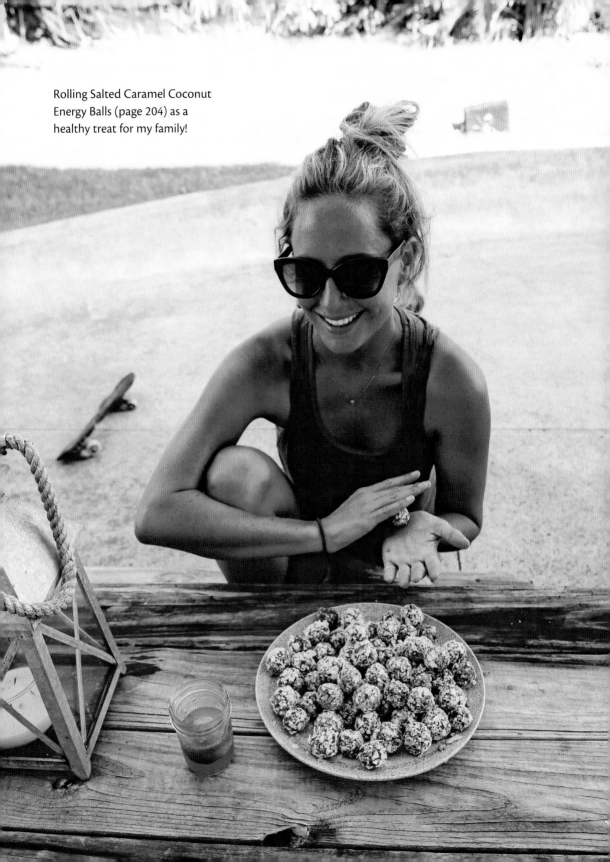

Rolling Salted Caramel Coconut Energy Balls (page 204) as a healthy treat for my family!

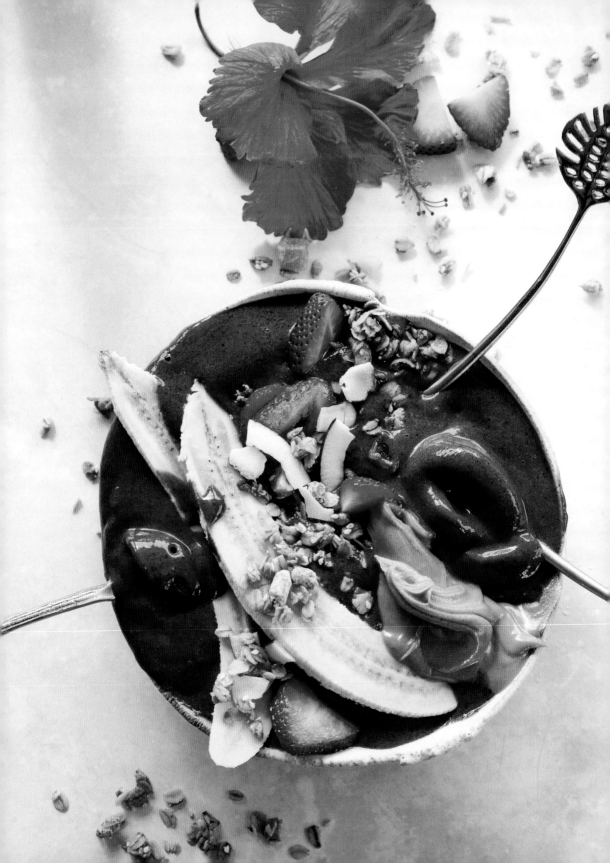

to your diet plan in a social setting in the chapters to come.

Four years later, my secret is out, and my entire family is predominantly plant-based. The number one rule in our home today is, you guessed it, "Plant Over Processed." This means that the majority of our diet is plants, and when we are hungry, we reach for something natural and plant-based before going for processed foods.

what can you expect from this book?

I want to make it as easy as possible for you to embrace a holistic, plant-based lifestyle. Throughout these pages, I'll help you to simplify your diet and your lifestyle in order to clear a path to better health. It will take some discipline to change your habits, as well as an open mind and the desire to learn. But I promise it will be fun, with plenty of easy-to-create, delicious recipes along the way!

We live in a time of abundance, when our dietary options are endless. This sounds positive, but if we're not careful, it can end up wreaking havoc on our health and causing confusion. Health issues linked to diet, like obesity, degenerative diseases, digestive issues, depression, and fatigue, are more prevalent today than at any other time in history, and they are controlling our lives. It is time to take a step back and look at the way we are living. Are you happy with the way that food is fueling your body? Or are you stressed out and making dietary decisions based on instant gratification, which in turn leads to a less happy and less healthy version of you?

My goal is to set you on a path toward better health by trusting nature, embracing balance, and using plant-based foods to nourish and fuel your body. Even if you don't suffer from the kinds of chronic health issues that I did, you can benefit immensely from following my Plant Over Processed rule as your mantra for healthy eating (and be sure to consult your doctor if you have concerns about particular health issues before making these changes, or any significant changes, to your diet).

Maybe you are thinking, "All of this is easy for you—you live in Hawaii!" Let me be the first to say that you don't need to be in Hawaii to live this lifestyle and to take care of yourself! There are affordable plant-based options everywhere, and the approach and recipes in this book are designed to work wherever you are. And wherever you are, remember to let nature lead the way. You can do this whether you live in a bustling city, in the suburbs, or near the beach. We will get into how to do this in the chapters to come!

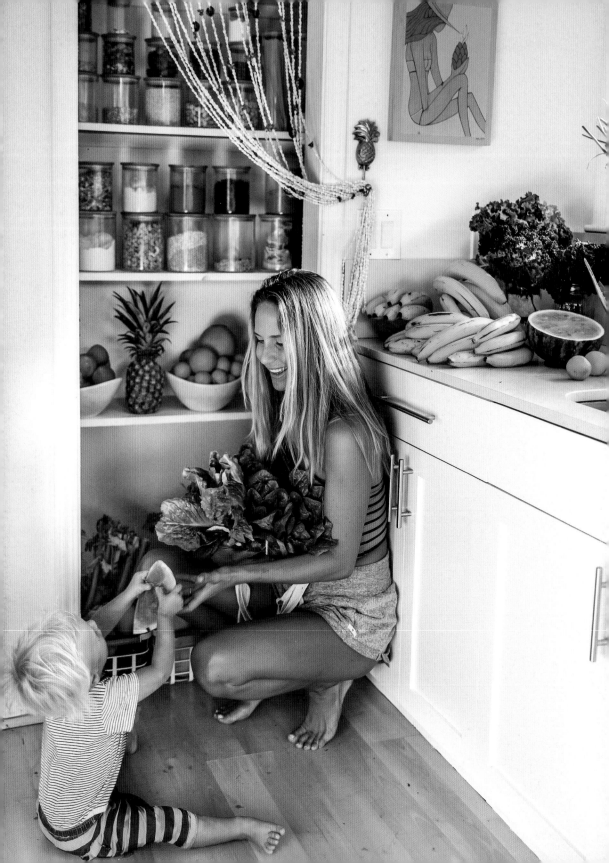

CHAPTER 1

the power of plants

One of the many beautiful things about following a plant-based diet is that this approach to eating comes with flexibility and it is meant to be personalized. Eating plant-based means feeding your body with nutrient-dense whole foods that are primarily (or entirely) derived from plants, with few (or no) animal products. Beyond that, the details are up to you. The goal is to find a way of eating that works for your body and that supports your lifestyle.

What that looks like will differ from one person to the next, and it could change for you over time. For example, if your goal right now is to add more plants to your diet, but you still want to eat fish on occasion, that's your choice. If you want to eat plant-based, but you don't want to give up real cheesecake, that's your choice too. You may want to continue to eat fish and cheesecake now and go completely vegan two years from now—that's great!

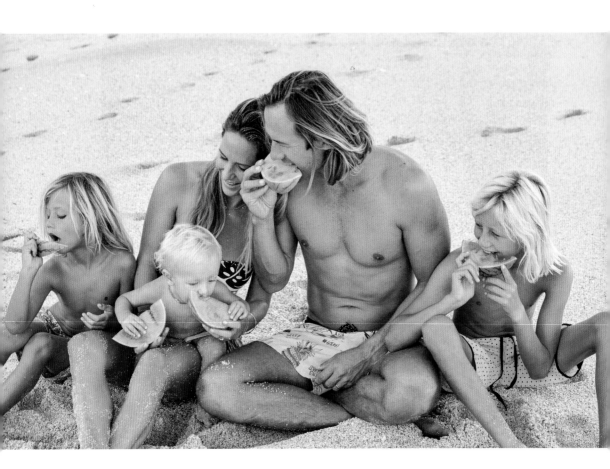

If you're reading this book, I'm going to assume that you are at least halfway there when it comes to signing on to the plant-based life. But in case you need a bit more convincing, here are the primary reasons why eating more plants will do your body good.

BETTER DIGESTION

A plant-centric diet is the best thing you can do for gut health. Plants are natural sources of fiber, which will keep you regular, eliminating bloat. Plants are also easier to digest than animal proteins and fats, eliminating many of the problems that those of us with sensitive digestive systems often deal with. It takes the body eighteen to twenty-four hours to break down and digest most meat, whereas fruits and vegetables take thirty to sixty minutes to digest and grains take around ninety minutes.

INCREASED ENERGY

If your body isn't spending time and effort on digestion, it has more energy to spend elsewhere. You might have noticed that more and more professional athletes are turning to plant-based diets. A big reason for this is because of how efficient the body becomes, not only during performance but also during healing from strenuous workouts and even injuries. Plants are also high in vitamins and minerals, which boost energy. And they are rich in antioxidants, phytonutrients, and the kinds of healthy fats, proteins, and carbs that make your body feel great.

WEIGHT LOSS

Do you know how many cups of broccoli you would need to eat to equal the number of calories in a palm-sized slice of cheesecake? Twenty-five! I know that broccoli might not sound as appealing to you as cheesecake, but my point is that you probably couldn't eat that much broccoli in an entire day, let alone in one sitting. Let's call this volume-based eating. Bottom line: Volume-based eating with plants means that you fill up more quickly and eat fewer calories, which naturally leads to weight loss.

Some people have concerns that the carbs in fruit, grains, and starches will make them gain weight. I totally get these concerns given the bad reputation that carbs have acquired in the health world. But really, the carbs you do want to avoid are refined carbs, which have been stripped of fiber and essentially contain empty calories, including sugar-sweetened drinks, fruit juices, pastries, and bleached flour products like crackers, cookies, and white bread. Good whole carbs are unprocessed and loaded with nutrients, protein, and fiber, and these include whole fruits and veggies, whole grains, potatoes, and legumes. You are more likely to lose unwanted weight than you are to gain following a plant-based and even high-carb diet.

MENTAL CLARITY AND HORMONAL BALANCE

I did not fully realize how foggy my brain was until I changed my diet. Before going plant-based, on a typical day I had a hard time collecting my thoughts and feeling in control of my emotions.

My body felt lifeless and tired and so did my mind. Besides feeling blah, I could tell my hormones were completely out of whack due to my menstrual cycle irregularities. For many years I would only get my period every six months or so and then, the year before I went plant-based, I was getting it every second week. This went on for almost seven months! I would get my period for seven days, have five to seven days off, and then it would start again. After months of this, I knew that something was truly off with my body.

A few weeks into my initial diet change, I remember feeling mentally clear and almost like a new person. I felt as if I was unlocking unused potential in myself. Two months into my diet change, my menstrual cycle became regular, and it has been regular ever since.

DISEASE PREVENTION

When I was fifteen, I was diagnosed with celiac disease, an immune reaction to eating gluten that can damage the small intestine and prevent the absorption of certain nutrients. Left unmanaged, celiac disease can lead to greater health complications over time. Several years later, I learned that I also had hypothyroidism, which is a dysfunction of the thyroid gland affecting nearly every part of the body, from the heart and brain to the muscles and skin. Untreated, hypothyroidism can lead to a host of awful symptoms, including changes in your menstrual cycle, constipation, depression, hair loss, dry skin,

and fatigue. I am fortunate that both were detected in time for me, and I have learned to manage my symptoms with a plant-based diet and the help of my doctor.

For those with celiac disease, going plant-based can help avoid flare-ups caused by accidentally eating something with gluten in it. Many sauces, processed foods, and meat fillers contain gluten, and eating plant-based has eliminated many of these problematic food choices for me. Like celiac disease, hypothyroidism is a chronic health issue, and the best way I have found to control mine is through a plant-based diet and exercise. I should note that for years I also took a small dose of levothyroxine for my hypothyroidism. I was told by doctors that this would be necessary long-term, but to my surprise and to my doctors' surprise, my blood tests recently came back showing that my thyroid is now functioning at a normal and healthy level. I no longer need medication! That's after four years of eating plant-based, and to me that's a huge testament to the power of eating this way.

Eating a plant-based diet may also reduce your risk of developing type 2 diabetes, heart disease, and cancer. Many experts also believe that a diet loaded with fruits and veggies prevents hypertension. I hope that you aren't dealing with anything close to the range of health issues that I was before going plant-based. But if you are concerned about any of the above, eating more plants can help in some very powerful ways.

the plant over processed lifestyle

I personally feel my absolute best when I adhere to a Plant Over Processed diet and the lifestyle that goes along with it. For me, this means getting 80 percent of my calories from high-volume living plant foods and 20 percent of my calories from cooked plant-based foods, with the occasional processed item. I get as close as I can to this ratio on a regular basis, and I don't keep close track of these percentages every day, although I did at first. I prefer to eat more intuitively now with this goal in mind. I would recommend tracking your goal percentages when you are just starting out until you fully get the hang of it. Keep in mind that your goals may be different than mine. Your aim may simply be to eat more plants—and that's great!

What I mean by high-volume living plant foods is plant foods that contain a large amount of water and fiber, such as all fruits and vegetables, as opposed to "low-volume" plant foods like nuts, seeds, grains, and plant-based oils. I consume low-volume plant foods sparingly, and I try to never fill myself up on them. This naturally keeps my diet low in fat and high in carbohydrates, and keeps me full, nourished, and satisfied. It also means I minimize my consumption of processed, fatty snack foods, including processed vegan snack foods that are labeled as healthy but that aren't really. Now that I know what it takes to stay strong and healthy, I can eat these foods sparingly and feel fine—and you may find this to be true for you too. But for the most part, I don't even want them because I have so many other delicious options in my diet.

When I first changed my diet in order to heal, I was very strict about what I would put into my body. For those first thirty days, I ate 100 percent vegan and nothing that was

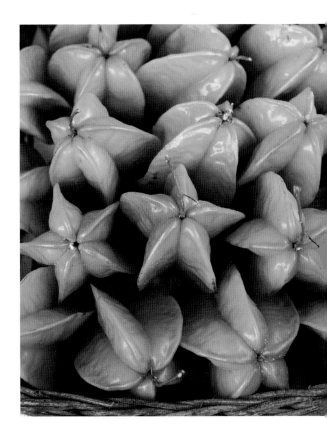

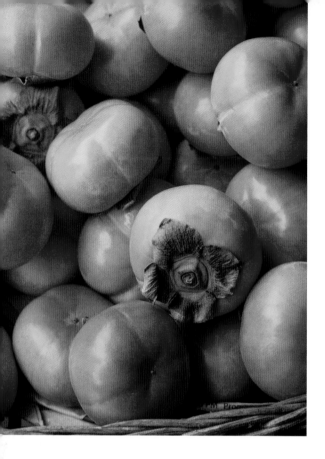

understand and experience the health and healing benefits of natural, plant-based foods and to help you develop a balanced lifestyle that is sustainable and that works for you!

Throughout this book I'll share my favorite plant-based recipes and dishes with you, but as a start, these are my favorite plant-based whole foods to prepare and cook with:

- **FRUITS:** I love whole fruits like mangos, bananas, apples, berries, pears, melons, peaches, grapes, dates, kiwis, lychees, limes, and lemons. I stay away from bottled fruit juice, as it often lacks nutrients and has added sugars.
- **VEGETABLES:** I eat starchy and non-starchy vegetables alike! My favorites are leafy greens, zucchini, cucumber, tomatoes, broccoli, fennel, potatoes, sweet potatoes, eggplant, peas, squash, and asparagus. Cruciferous vegetables like broccoli, cauliflower, and cabbage are best eaten cooked, as they can be hard to digest and cause gas when consumed raw. For the same reason, kale and Swiss chard are also better cooked or blended in a smoothie.
- **WHOLE GRAINS:** My favorite whole grains are gluten-free oats, brown rice, quinoa, amaranth, and millet. I stay away from processed, refined flours but do eat white rice on occasion.
- **SEEDS AND SPROUTS:** I love omega-3-fatty-acid-rich sunflower seeds, chia

processed or that contained added chemicals or preservatives. I also ate raw for my first two meals of the day, to ensure I was nourishing my body with natural living foods. I needed an extreme change to reset my body, but today I am much more lenient about what I eat. I even indulge on special occasions and still feel great. As I've mentioned, plant-based is meant to be personalized. Our bodies are all different and we all have different health needs and goals. In this chapter I will share what works for me and for my family, but you can tailor and adjust as necessary to meet your needs. There are so many ways to interpret this lifestyle. My goal is to help you

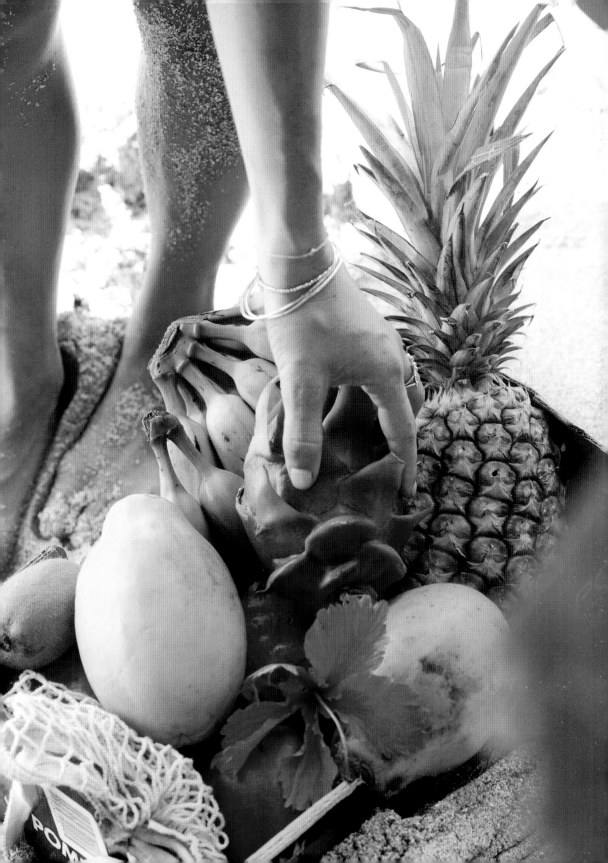

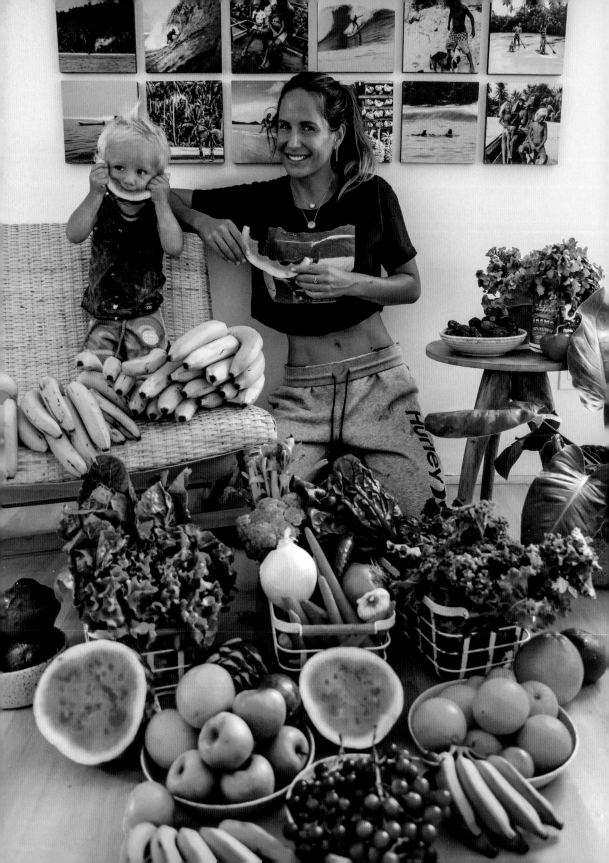

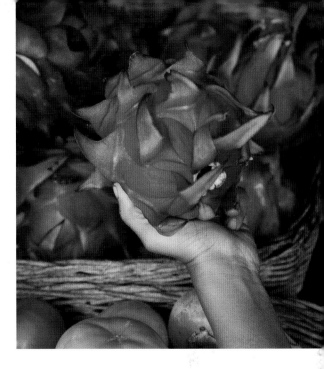

seeds, flaxseeds, and hemp seeds. Great sprouts include pumpkin sprouts, bean sprouts, and horseradish sprouts.

- **HERBS AND SPICES:** These are all fair game! Use any fresh herb or dried spice to add flavor to your food, including mixed blends like chili powder, garam masala, curry powder, and pumpkin spice, as well as cumin, onion powder, paprika, bay leaf, black pepper, turmeric, lemon pepper, cilantro, basil, parsley, mint, and chives.

- **SOY PRODUCTS:** Tofu, tempeh, and edamame are excellent sources of healthy protein and easy to add to recipes.

- **LEGUMES AND NUTS:** Lentils, chickpeas, hazelnuts, almonds, Brazil nuts, cashews, macadamia nuts, and nuts and legumes of all kinds are excellent sources of protein, fiber, and healthy fats.

- **BEVERAGES:** Water is your OG beverage that's going to support you every day for life, but herbal teas, smoothies, and cold-pressed green juices are great choices too.

- **OILS:** Organic extra virgin olive oil is my favorite healthy oil.

- **SWEETENERS:** Agave nectar, dates, coconut sugar, and maple syrup are all great natural choices for sweetening your food. Avoid refined sugars as much as possible, along with artificial sweeteners.

There are so many ways to enjoy these fresh, delicious whole foods, whether combined in recipes or on their own. To me there is nothing more delicious than biting into a crunchy, sweet apple, or digging into a whole avocado sprinkled with a bit of sea salt and a squeeze of lime. If these sound boring to you, it may be because your taste buds have been desensitized by a diet of processed foods and refined sugars. You need to give your brain and your tongue some time to reacclimate! Every two weeks or so our taste buds change—they expire and regenerate like any other cells in the body. This means that we can retrain our palates to prefer more natural tastes—with their built-in nutritional benefits—as opposed to the high sugar, high salt, chemically laced tastes that we may be accustomed to.

is plant-based the same as vegan?

According to the Vegan Society, veganism is "a way of living which seeks to exclude, as far as is possible and practicable, all forms of exploitation of, and cruelty to, animals for food, clothing or any other purpose." Strict vegans do not consume or wear animal products, and many avoid products that have been tested on animals. There is a lot of overlap between plant-based and vegan lifestyles, but the two approaches are not synonymous. Veganism is a serious title to wear, and for many it is a moral decision. While I have the utmost respect for veganism, it's a lifestyle that does not come with a lot of wiggle room. The plant-based approach is a better fit for me because it entails being mindful of my food choices and their effects on an ethical scale, with a focus on plant-based foods. It's also important to keep in mind that it is entirely possible to eat vegan without really eating healthy, if the bulk of your diet comes from vegan junk foods like cookies, cakes, and processed carbohydrates. You can technically be vegan and live on Oreos, but this is not the plant-based lifestyle!

what your body needs

Is it possible to get all the nutrients that your body needs from plants? The answer is: Yes! Perhaps this comes as a surprise, but the truth is that fueling and nourishing your body with plants is no more difficult than maintaining a healthy diet that includes animal products. The first step is to educate yourself so that you know what your body needs and understand how certain foods work in the body. Let's take a look at what healthy eating and nourishing your body are all about, with a little help from Oahu-based naturopathic physician Dr. Diana Joy Ostroff. Dr. Ostroff has been an invaluable resource throughout my health journey, and she has vetted and approved all of the health information in this book.

Before you embark on your new plant-based eating plan or make any major dietary change, I recommend consulting your doctor and going in for a checkup and routine bloodwork.

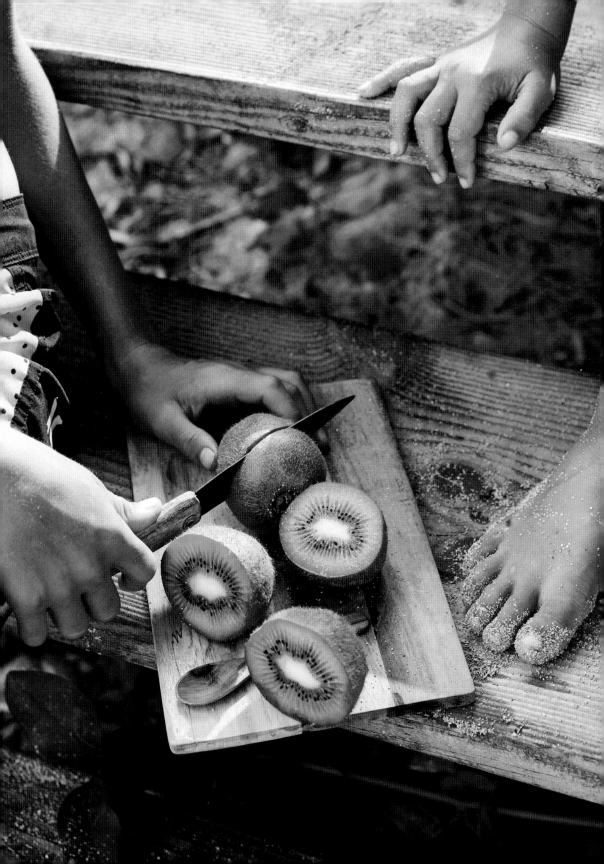

healthy fats

Healthy fats not only help your body to absorb important fat-soluble nutrients, they also help your body on a cellular level. Healthy fats protect your cells from damage, acting like a lubricating cushion for them. Healthy fats can be found in a variety of plant-based foods, including nuts, seeds, olive oil, flaxseed oil, avocados, and cacao nibs. Use oils sparingly, as excess oil can be hard to digest. I personally like to use high-quality olive oil and cold-pressed flaxseed oil in my recipes.

When we talk about "healthy fats," we're referring to monounsaturated fats (found in olive oil, avocados, and certain nuts) and polyunsaturated fats (found in seeds and nuts, as well as fish oils and oysters), as opposed to saturated fats (found in butter, dairy, and many animal products). Consuming plant-based fats lowers LDL cholesterol (the "bad" kind of cholesterol) and helps to reduce inflammation (which has been linked to heart disease, stroke, and cancer), while animal fats and hydrogenated oils with high trans fats can raise LDL cholesterol and cause inflammation. Oils rich in monounsaturated fats also contain vitamin E, which is a powerful antioxidant. Polyunsaturated fats contain omega-3 fatty acids, which have been proved to be beneficial for heart health.

vitamins

There are thirteen essential vitamins that your body needs to function. Our bodies produce some of these vitamins naturally, and others we need to get from the foods we eat.

VITAMIN B_{12}

Vitamin B_{12} is important for the development of our brain, nervous system, and the production of red blood cells. B_{12} deficiency can lead to anemia, digestive issues, and nerve damage, which is why it's important to get your proper dose. The body does not produce vitamin B_{12} on its own, and B_{12} does not exist in plants. Certain animal products (including beef, liver, chicken, fish, and shellfish) are rich in B_{12}, but if you are following a plant-based diet, B_{12} is also easy and inexpensive to get in the form of a pill, a B_{12} shot from a health lab, or from fortified cereals or other fortified foods. However you get it, just make sure that you do, as it will support your health efforts!

VITAMIN D

Vitamin D is essential for building and maintaining strong, healthy bones because your body cannot absorb calcium without the presence of vitamin D. There is debate within the scientific community about exactly how much vitamin D your body needs, but experts all agree that it is one of the most important vitamins. Ideally, we would get all the vitamin D that we need from the sun, but if you live in a place where you don't get regular sun exposure (at least fifteen minutes a day, without sunscreen), if

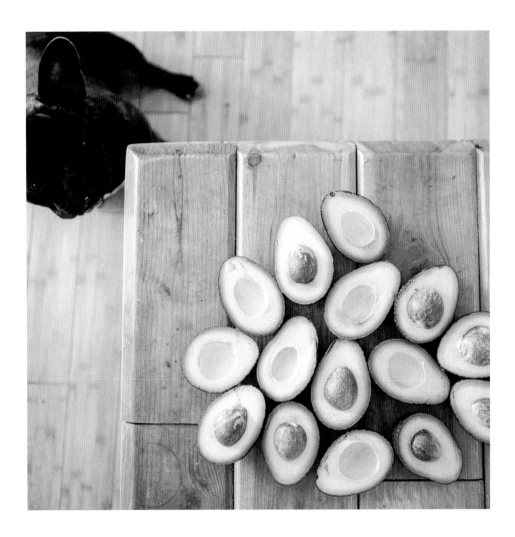

your skin is dark (the more melanin in your skin, the longer it takes for your body to produce vitamin D from the sun), or if you are over sixty-five, take a vitamin D supplement to cover your bases. You can also get vitamin D through plant-based foods including mushrooms, fortified soy milk, and fortified almond milk.

protein

We need protein to keep our skin, bones, muscles, and organs healthy. The amount you need changes with age, and there is some disagreement among experts on exact amounts, but the current Recommended Dietary Allowance (RDA) for protein is 0.36 gram of protein per pound of body weight.

So, for a person who weighs 140 pounds, that's about 50 grams per day. If you have concerns about your protein requirements, consult your doctor.

The good news is that it is easy for most everyone, including vegetarians and vegans, to meet their daily protein requirements. Protein is present in both plant and animal products, and you may be surprised by how quickly the seemingly small amounts of protein in plants can add up. There are a number of reasons to choose plant protein over animal protein. From a health perspective, there is evidence to suggest that diets high in animal protein are linked to various types of cancer, as well as to heart disease and diabetes. I personally don't track the exact amounts of protein I'm consuming, but I make sure to eat a variety of plant-based proteins. I like to give my smoothies a burst of extra protein by adding plant protein powder. (My favorite is Pure Vegan Pea Protein, and I recommend choosing a protein powder made with simple, plant-based ingredients with no additives or flavorings.) I'll also add a spoonful of hemp hearts, a dollop of nut butter, and/or chia seeds to my smoothies for extra protein. Here is a list of some great plant-based protein sources:

LENTILS (COOKED): 18 grams per cup
BEANS: black beans, kidney beans, chickpeas, pinto beans, and lima beans (cooked)—15 grams per cup

EDAMAME (COOKED): 17 grams per cup
TEMPEH: 31 grams per cup
SEITAN: 21 grams per 3-ounce serving
TOFU: 11 grams per 4-ounce serving
SPINACH (COOKED): 5 grams per cup
BROCCOLI (COOKED): 4 grams per cup
QUINOA (COOKED): 8 grams per cup
PEAS (COOKED): 8 grams per cup
ALMONDS: 8 grams per ¼ cup

minerals

The minerals that we need to pay the most attention to in our diets are calcium, iron, iodine, and zinc. And you can get all of these minerals from whole, plant-based foods! Let's take a look at each one individually to get a feel for their importance, where to get them, and how to make sure we are getting enough.

IRON

Iron is an essential nutrient for many functions in the body, including transporting oxygen throughout our bodies via red blood cells. Iron-rich plant sources include dark leafy greens, quinoa, legumes, lentils, enriched cereals, and prunes. Recommended iron intakes vary depending on your age and gender (young children and women who are pregnant or have their periods are at higher risk for iron deficiency).

When following a plant-based diet, it is important to understand that there are two types of iron: heme iron, which is found in meat, and non-heme iron, which is found in plants. Non-heme iron is not absorbed in the body as efficiently as heme iron. However, despite the lower absorption rate, most vegetarians and vegans consume enough iron. As a rule of thumb, people who do not consume animal products need twice as much iron as people who do. The daily recommendation for a non-vegan adult man between nineteen and fifty years old is 8 mg, and it's 18 mg for a woman of the same age. For those not eating meat, the numbers should be doubled.

TIP: You can increase your iron absorption rate by consuming foods high in vitamin C (cantaloupe, oranges, berries, watermelon, mango, papaya, and grapefruit) with your iron sources. Drink coffee and tea or take calcium supplements only between meals, as these slow iron absorption.

CALCIUM

Calcium does a lot—it builds healthy bones and teeth, keeps your heart beating, prevents your blood from clotting, and allows your muscles to contract. We get calcium through the foods we eat, and good plant-based sources of calcium include dark green leafy vegetables like kale, spinach, bok choy, parsley, broccoli, and collard greens; nori (dried edible seaweed); almonds; and sesame seeds. Blackstrap molasses and fortified drinks like orange juice, soy milk, and almond milk also contain calcium, as do edamame and tofu.

The recommended daily dose of calcium for a woman under fifty is 1,000 mg, and for age fifty and older it's 1,200 mg. For a man under seventy the recommended daily dose is 1,000 mg, and for age seventy and older it's 1,200 mg daily. Also, as mentioned, you need adequate levels of vitamin D in your body to absorb calcium.

ZINC

Zinc helps the immune system defend against bacteria and viruses. It also assists the body in making proteins and DNA, helps wounds heal, and is important for proper taste and smell. Zinc is important, but we only need a small amount on a daily basis (8 mg for women, 11 mg for men). Plant-based sources of zinc are soy products, spinach, nuts, seeds, wheat germ, beans, mushrooms, grains, and legumes. Soaking legumes and sprouting grains are the best choices and can increase the absorption of zinc!

IODINE

We rely on iodine to make thyroid hormones, which control the body's metabolism and regulate the growth and function of key organs. Americans are rarely iodine deficient because just ¼ teaspoon of iodized salt daily provides a significant amount of iodine. But if

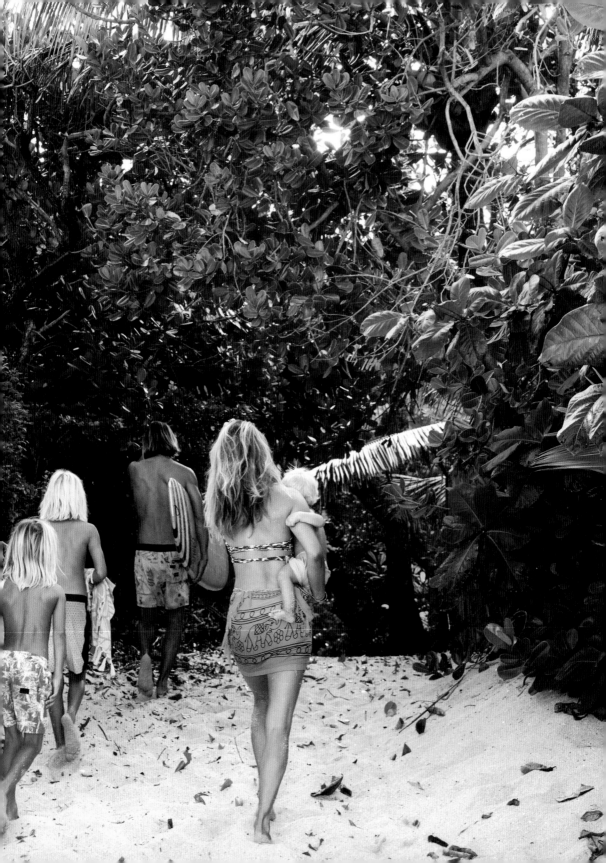

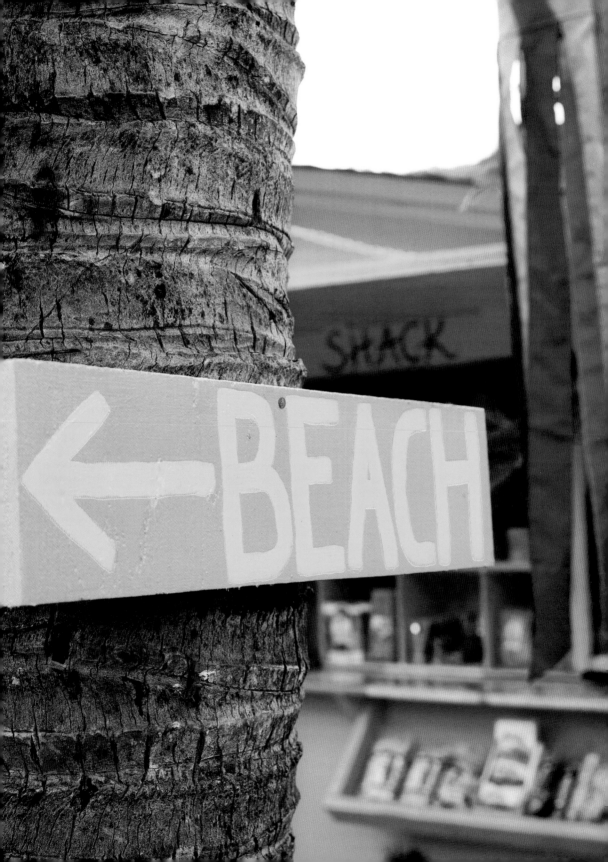

you exclusively use sea salt or another fancy salt that isn't iodized, make sure you are getting iodine somewhere else. Seaweed is a great source!

sugar!

Sugar is not a nutrient, and most of us are consuming too much of it—particularly the refined kind. There is a big difference between the kind of refined sugar found in donuts and the naturally occurring sugar found in fruits and other plants. The body recognizes and processes these sugars differently, which can affect your overall health. Natural sugars are digested more slowly, helping you to feel full for longer while keeping your metabolism stable. Refined sugars on the other hand are broken down quickly by the body, causing insulin and blood sugar levels to spike, and leaving you craving more sugar, no matter how much you've consumed.

For years I was a total refined sugar junkie: Mars Bars, Cocoa Puffs, and Cap'n Crunch were some of my favorites. Often these foods were my meals! My body felt terrible when I was eating this way, and I tried to quit sugar again and again, without success. I'm not the only one who has struggled with this issue. While the American Heart Association recommends no more than 6 teaspoons (25 grams) of added/refined sugar per day for women, and 9 teaspoons (38 grams) for men, the average American consumes around 20 teaspoons a day! We

are a nation of sugar addicts. The processed foods that we eat are in large part to blame. Many of us are having dessert three times a day without even realizing it. (Hello, Zucchini Walnut Muffin from Starbucks with 500 calories and almost 30 grams of sugar.) Sugar consumption has been linked to an increased risk of cardiovascular disease, type 2 diabetes, cancer, tooth decay, anxiety, and obesity, along with premature aging, which is why it is important to get that sweet tooth under control.

Don't beat yourself up if you are feeling out of control with your sugar cravings. Sugar is actually considered an addictive substance with druglike effects on the brain. Researchers have found that eating something sweet can activate pleasure centers in the brain, causing the release of dopamine, the chemical that causes feelings of pleasure and happiness. The same thing happens with the anticipation of a sweet treat. Our brains get hooked on this "pleasure and reward" cycle, which leaves us craving more, with our sweet tooth getting increasingly harder to satiate. And we are constantly tempted—if you are a sugar addict, every time you pass a bakery or see an ad for Cinnabon, this response gets activated!

It doesn't help that 80 percent of foods on the supermarket shelf have added sugar. We live in a world where food companies have figured out that by adding more sugar to their products, even if they aren't meant to be sweet, they can keep us hooked. The tastier a packaged convenience food is, the more profitable it is, because we keep coming back for more. How do we break this cycle?

1. **UNDERSTAND HOW SUGAR AFFECTS THE BODY, AND WHY YOU CRAVE IT.** The more aware you are, the better equipped you will be to make healthy choices.

2. **BELIEVE THAT IT'S POSSIBLE TO CHANGE.** You can begin to reprogram your habits and your cravings in one to two weeks, by training your taste buds and your brain to respond to real, whole foods as opposed to the sugary, processed stuff. You can also learn to delay gratification and to associate pleasurable eating with the preparation of a healthy dinner, rather than with reaching for a processed convenience food.

3. **PREPARE FOR TEMPTATION AND HAVE HEALTHY ALTERNATIVES AVAILABLE.** The recipes that I'm going to share with you in this book are great, healthy options that contain little or no processed sugar. These will be your greatest assets in fighting those sugar cravings.

Now that you've got the basics, it's time to start building new healthy habits. Your taste buds are going to change, and so will your body as you begin to make the connection between what you are eating and how it makes you feel. This is an exciting place to be, so believe in the process, and know that it *can* become second nature to go for plant over processed when you are hungry!

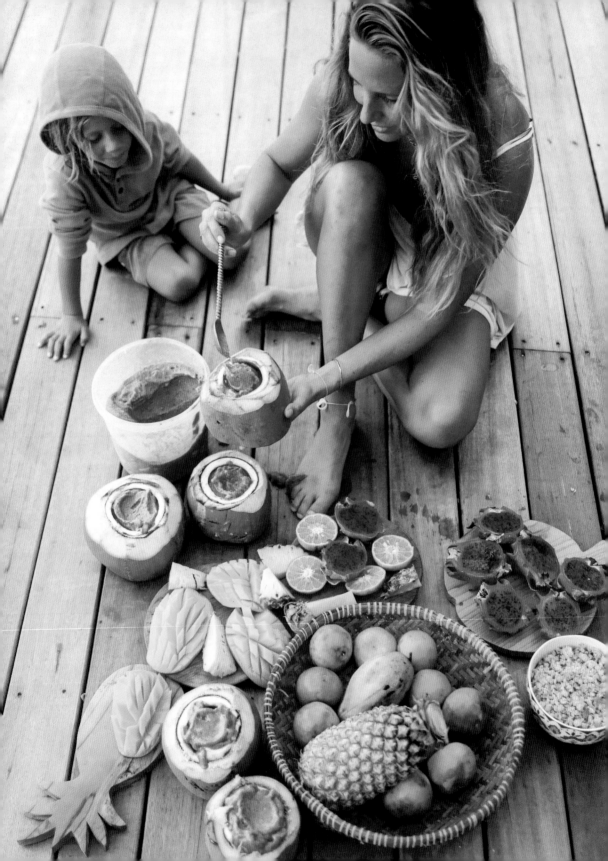

CHAPTER 2

the 30-day plant over processed challenge

When I first made the commitment to change the way I was eating and to eat 100 percent plant-based for thirty days, I decided to hold off on judging whether this diet was "working" for me until the thirty days were over. I recommend that you do the same, as your body and your mind will need those thirty days to adjust and adapt, and to build new healthy habits. After my thirty-day challenge, I couldn't believe how great I felt. I never looked back! I hope that you will have the same experience.

It's important to keep in mind, however, that change doesn't happen overnight. You will most likely experience an uncomfortable transition period as your body detoxes.

Welcome these symptoms because they are signs that your body is changing, cleaning house, and evolving into the healthier, more fabulous version of you! You may initially experience headaches, cravings, and breakouts, or feel sluggish, moody, or just a little off. Your detox symptoms may last anywhere from a few days to a few weeks, depending on the state of your health when you begin this challenge. When I initially did this detox, for the first two to three weeks I felt more bloated than usual (a sign that my gut was detoxing), I had withdrawal headaches, and experienced skin issues. It wasn't an enjoyable period, but it was a small price to pay for what was next: vibrant health from the inside out.

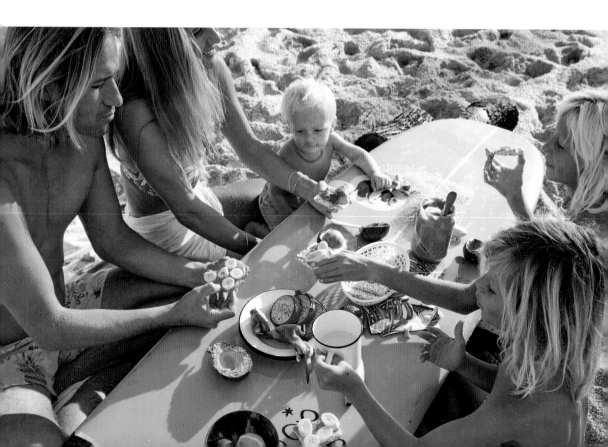

the challenge

Okay, it's time to get started! These are the ground rules for your 30-Day Plant Over Processed Challenge, followed by guidelines for each of the three individual phases of this detox.

the rules

1. **THE GOLDEN RULE:** For each meal that you eat during your 30-Day Challenge, 80 percent of your calories will come from living, or predominantly living, plant-based, whole foods, and the other 20 percent will come from cooked plant-based foods.

2. **PLANT OVER PROCESSED:** Avoid processed foods at all costs. I can't stress this enough. Whole foods will heal, detox, and rejuvenate your body during this period.

3. **CUT OUT REFINED SUGAR:** We've covered the harms of added sugar already (see page 26). Eliminate the white stuff. Enough said.

4. **AVOID CAFFEINE, ALCOHOL, AND ARTIFICIAL SWEETENERS:** The idea here isn't to torture you, but to retrain your body and your mind to function without these things. If this is too extreme, opt for natural over artificial— coffee or tea over energy drinks and diet sodas. Otherwise, drink water, and lots of it, along with herbal teas and your Digestion-Boosting Morning Tonic (page 35).

5. **IF YOU ARE HUNGRY, EAT!** Don't worry about portion control or restricting calories when eating high-volume plant foods.

6. **EAT RAW UNTIL DINNER:** During this challenge period, make the first two meals of the day predominantly or completely raw. Breakfast may be a Digestion-Boosting Morning Tonic (page 35) followed by a nourishing green smoothie. Lunch may be a big green salad with fruit, veggies, and nuts.

7. **END THE DAY WITH A HOT, NOURISHING PLANT-BASED MEAL:** During this period, it's great to make dinner a cooked plant-based meal— perhaps a soup or curry, a vegan stir-fry, or a roasted veggie burrito. I recommend adding a side salad along with dinner as well.

8. **CHOOSE FROM MY FAVORITES:** To make things as easy as possible, go for the breakfast, lunch, dinner, dessert, and snack options that I've provided for you in the next chapter. These recipes are my tried-and-true favorites—I make them all on

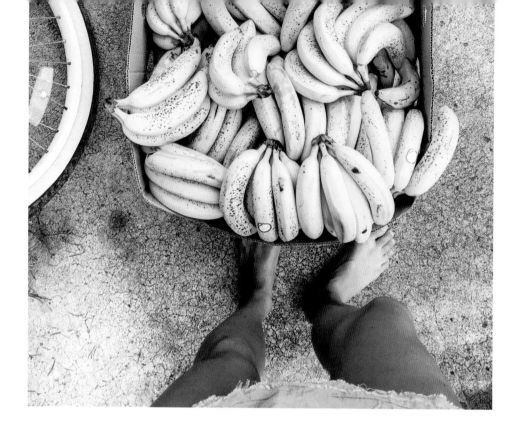

a regular basis for myself and my family, because they are incredibly easy and delicious! The recipes in the chapter that follows are categorized under:

LIVING PLANT-BASED RECIPE

PREDOMINANTLY LIVING PLANT-BASED RECIPE

COOKED PLANT-BASED RECIPE

to make it easier for you to follow my 80/20 Rule.

9. **PRACTICE FOOD COMBINING:** Food combining is a way of eating rooted in the ancient practice of Ayurveda, based on the idea that certain foods pair well together, while others do not. I practice a modified approach to food combining, and eat certain foods together depending on the amount of time they take to digest. See more on how food combining works in the box opposite.

10. **IT'S NOT ABOUT PERFECTION:** If you get off track for whatever reason, do not worry! The 30-Day Challenge is not about punishing yourself. The ultimate goal is to establish a positive relationship with plant-based foods and to experience the benefits of eating more plants. This is not a diet—it's a new way of thinking about the way that you eat, and whether what you are eating is making you feel your best.

FOOD COMBINING

Food combining is an approach to eating based on the concept that certain food combinations are easier to digest than others. The goal of food combining is to eat in a way that aids digestion and increases the nutrients your body absorbs. In my experience, food combining is one of the most effective ways to improve the digestive process, control gas and bloating, and increase energy. If you have a sensitive digestive system, this practice can make a big difference in your daily life.

There are a number of approaches to food combining, many of them complicated, but I am going to simplify things for you here, for plant-based eating. For starters, I follow these simple principles:

1. Throughout the course of the day, eat foods in the order of how long they take to digest, with the foods that take the least time to digest earlier in the day and slower-digesting foods later in the day.
2. If a given meal includes a variety of food groups, you can improve your digestion by working around your plate in the order of how fast each food digests, fastest to slowest.

So how quickly do various foods digest?

- Melons are best first thing in the morning on an empty stomach, as they are the fastest digesting food. Digestion time: approximately five to ten minutes.
- All other fruits are the second fastest digesting foods and are best eaten before cooked foods if eaten during the same meal. Digestion time: approximately thirty minutes. (Rule of thumb: Eat fruits before cooked foods unless you wait three to four hours in between.)
- Greens and raw vegetables are considered "neutral" and can be paired with any food group to assist in the digestion process.
- Cooked foods—legumes, grains, and starchy vegetables—are the third fastest digesting foods, and therefore should be eaten last if following a plant-based diet. This is why I prefer to make my first two meals of the day raw on a regular basis.
- If you are not following a vegan diet, note that meat takes the most time to digest, eighteen to twenty-four hours, or even longer. I found a huge increase in my energy levels after eliminating meat from my diet, and I credit it to how much less energy my body is spending on digestion.
- For additional information on avoiding bloat and aiding digestion, see Phase One Guideposts (page 36).

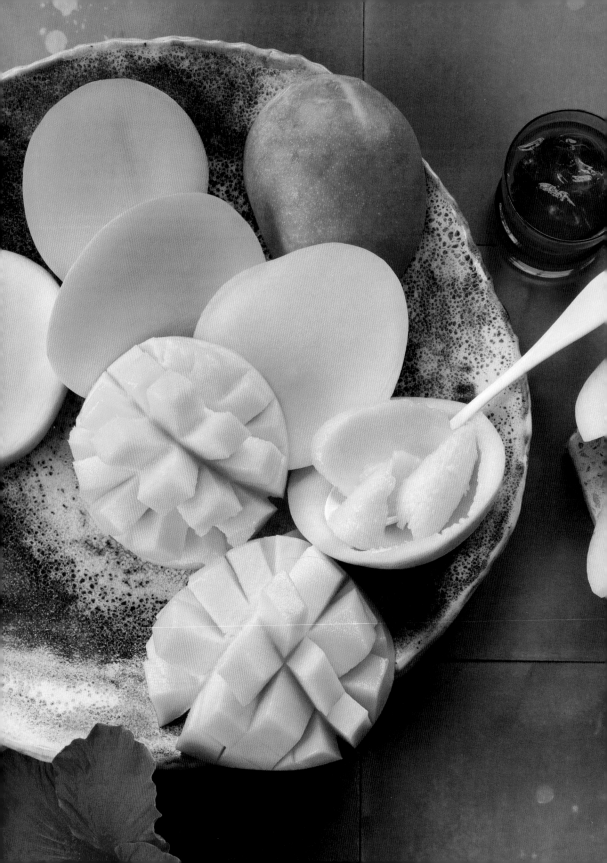

MAKE IT A MONO MEAL FOR BETTER DIGESTION

A "Mono Meal" is a meal made up of one type of fruit; you eat just that fruit for a meal until you are full. Eating this way can ease digestion if you have an unsettled stomach. Fruits that work best as Mono Meals are melons for breakfast (because these are easiest on the digestive system), as well as bananas, mangos, and oranges. When I first changed my diet, I started to regularly incorporate Mono Meals a few times a week, and eating this way did wonders for me! Today I go for a Mono Meal whenever I need a bit of a digestion boost. I also like to include a side of tender leafy greens like baby spinach, or a side of celery, with a Mono Meal as a way to add extra fiber, vitamins, and minerals while allowing the glucose in the fruit to be released even more slowly and evenly.

digestion-boosting morning tonic

PREP TIME: 5 MINUTES • TOTAL TIME: 5 MINUTES • SERVES 1

One of the most powerful things you can do for your health is to drink lots of water and stay hydrated! Start first thing in the morning with this tonic, which contains cayenne pepper to boost your metabolism and lemon juice to cleanse your system.

1 cup filtered water
Juice of 1 lemon
1 teaspoon maple syrup, or to taste
1 pinch cayenne pepper

Mix all the ingredients together in a glass and enjoy over ice, at room temperature, or hot like a tea.

phase one: the jump-start

days 1–10

You're pumped! You're ready to change your body and your life, and to start each morning with a tonic and a nourishing smoothie, rather than biting into dessert disguised as breakfast (aka a sugary muffin). Warning: You will need to hold tightly to that early enthusiasm as you progress through this journey, because the waters may get rough. Most people who clean up their diet encounter hangover-like symptoms, including headaches, fatigue, brain fog, bloat, and overall moodiness. By day two or three of your detox, you may even notice that your tongue has a white coating and that no matter how many times you brush your teeth, your mouth never feels clean. Believe it or not, these are signs of progress. These symptoms are signs that your body is detoxing, releasing impurities that have built up over years of unhealthful choices.

Hang in there. As your body detoxes and begins to adjust to your new way of eating, these symptoms will eventually dissipate. If you still feel like you want to punch a wall by day five, remind yourself that there is a lot going on for you at this moment. Not only is your body trying to figure out how to handle these new foods coming in, it is wondering when the old, familiar processed food is

coming back. You may find yourself wanting to fall back into old, familiar habits. Resist the urge! Right now, your brain and your body are in conflict, and they will just have to agree to disagree. But soon, very soon, they will be on the same page about all of the healthy new foods that are coming in. Just give it a bit more time!

PHASE ONE GUIDEPOSTS

- Start each day of Phase One with a Digestion-Boosting Morning Tonic (page 35), followed by breakfast, lunch, dinner, snack, and dessert options from Chapter 3.
- Make batches of your favorite Earth Bowl dressings (pages 186–189) at the beginning of the week to use in meals throughout the week. At the start of the week, make extras of a few recipes that you can store as leftovers for the rest of the week. For example, if you are making one of the soups, double the recipe and freeze half. If you are roasting veggies, make extra to add as a side to dinners throughout the week.
- During Phase One, practice food combining for optimal digestion,

particularly if you have a sensitive digestive system. The idea behind food combining is that you eat certain foods together, or avoid eating certain foods together, depending on the amount of time they take to digest. Since fruits are the fastest and easiest foods to digest, breakfast should be a smoothie or fruit on its own, as a Mono Meal (see page 35). For lunch, try a big salad (see pages 117–121), a smoothie (see pages 69–80), or an Earth Bowl (see pages 105–114). For dinner, try a soup or curry (see pages 143–157) or one of my other plant-based meals (see pages 125–141).

- Avoid the following bloat-sensitive plant foods during this phase:
  - Raw vegetables that cause gas— broccoli, kale, cabbage, cauliflower, asparagus, mushrooms, and Brussels sprouts. Eating these vegetables cooked is okay.
  - Raw or cooked garlic.
  - Raw onion. Cooked or pickled onions are great—pickled onion can actually aid digestion.
- Throughout Phase One, get plenty of exercise and move your body as much as possible. Do whatever form of exercise you love, whether that's walking, running, taking a fitness class, or practicing yoga.

PHYSICAL SYMPTOMS TO EXPECT DURING PHASE ONE

- Headaches
- Fatigue
- Brain fog
- Bloating
- Moodiness

BENEFITS THAT YOU ARE WORKING TOWARD

- Improved digestion
- Increased energy
- Weight loss or maintenance
- Muscle tone
- Heightened mental clarity (no more brain fog)
- Hormonal balance/a feeling of stability
- Clearer skin, whiter eyes, shinier hair, stronger nails
- Satisfied feeling after every meal and no more cravings (Note: If you are still craving salt, fats, or sweets, it is usually a sign that you are not eating enough carbohydrates—fruit—throughout the day.)
- No need for stimulants such as coffee

phase two: making waves

days 11–20

The start of Phase Two may be when you hit a wall and decide that Plant Over Processed isn't going to work for you. Or you could be feeling unstoppable. It all depends on your starting point. Again, hang in there! Your body is still learning to adapt to this new way of eating, and it is figuring out how to repair the damage done by your old, processed diet.

Be patient, trust the process, and remember that the nutritious food you are consuming is restoring your gut and your body. If you are feeling bored or isolated, try inviting some friends over for a plant-based potluck. Other strategies to get you through this period include treating yourself to a massage or going on a special hike to celebrate the amazing things you are doing for your body. If you also need to scream into a pillow, do it! It's cathartic.

PHASE TWO GUIDEPOSTS

- During Phase Two, detox symptoms may dissipate or diminish completely, and you may start to feel the rewards of improved energy, digestion, and mental clarity. If this hasn't happened yet, remember that it may take longer to feel positive results, depending on where you were health-wise when you started this challenge.
- Start each day of Phase Two with your Digestion-Boosting Morning Tonic (page 35), and feel free to drink this same

elixir between meals to hydrate, aid the cleansing process, and curb cravings and hunger.

- Enjoy breakfast, lunch, dinner, snack, and dessert options from Chapter 3, no longer avoiding the bloat-sensitive foods listed for Phase One (see page 37) if bloating hasn't been an issue thus far.
- Follow the food combining principles outlined under Phase One (see page 33), and eat until satisfied with each meal, without restricting or counting calories. You might find yourself wanting to eat a lot, and that's okay! Dive into a massive Earth Bowl and enjoy every bite. Don't let yourself go hungry or it will get harder to stay on track.
- Continue supporting your transformation efforts with exercise! Move your body as much as possible, in whatever way makes you feel great.

PHYSICAL SYMPTOMS TO EXPECT DURING PHASE TWO

- Depending on your personal health state going into this challenge, you may continue to experience some or all of the Phase One detox symptoms.
- You may also be experiencing some of the future benefits listed under Phase One (see page 37).

phase three: a whole new you

days 21–30

The first few days of Phase Three are when you will begin to notice your cravings subside if you haven't already, along with the extra bloat, moodiness, and fatigue. By the start of Phase Three, you are probably also feeling more confident about shopping for groceries, and you will have mastered many of the plant-based recipes in this book. With that said, after twenty-plus days of eating this way, you may be feeling bored and restricted, or longing for your old comfort foods. If this becomes the case for you, remember that what feels restrictive now is the key to unlocking your freedom from cravings, fatigue, brain fog, skin issues, digestive issues, and unwanted weight. Keep your eye on the prize: getting to the end of your 30-Day Challenge. This process will not only strengthen and heal your body, it will strengthen your character. I am rooting for you!

PHASE THREE GUIDEPOSTS

- During Phase Three, your body will emerge from the transitional phase of the detox, and you will begin to experience the full, energizing, transformative effects of Plant Over Processed:
  - Increased energy
  - Weight loss or maintenance
  - Muscle tone
  - Heightened mental clarity (no more brain fog)
  - Feeling satisfied after every meal (no more cravings)
  - No need for stimulants such as coffee
  - Hormonal balance/a feeling of stability
  - Clearer skin, whiter eyes, shinier hair, stronger nails

- Continue to drink your Digestion-Boosting Morning Tonic (page 35) in the morning and between meals as desired.
- Continue to eat breakfast, lunch, dinner, dessert, and snacks by choosing from the recipes in Chapter 3.
- Over the course of Phase Three, gradually begin to personalize your Plant Over Processed eating plan to reflect your needs, lifestyle, and goals. This means that if there are certain non-plant-based foods, or certain processed foods that you want to enjoy on occasion, you can begin eating them again in moderation. As you phase these foods back in, pay careful attention to how your body responds, to be sure that eating these items is really what's best for you!

you made it! now what?

When you get to the end of your 30-Day Challenge, give yourself a major pat on the back. Sticking to your guns took some serious self-discipline. You rock! In addition to feeling the benefits listed above, you may also notice that food tastes different now—you may no longer crave some of the things that you once did, or you may like foods that you never did before! This is because the 30-Day Challenge is a total reset that cleanses your system and puts you back in touch with your body's internal cues. What do I mean by internal cues? I mean the messages that your body is sending you about what it *really* needs to feel great. When your body is hopped up on sugar and processed junk, you may think it is telling you that you *need cheesecake right now*. But after you eliminate these toxins from your system, your body will finally be able to tell you which foods it actually needs and which it doesn't. Congratulations! This is a powerful place to be.

So what's next? Do you eat this way forever? At the end of my challenge I felt so fantastic that I wanted to keep it up. I stuck to my 80/20 Rule and I continued to eat raw or predominantly raw for my first two meals of the day, followed by a cooked plant-based meal for dinner. I opted for Plant Over Processed whenever I could, and this is the

way that I eat today. Hopefully at this point you are feeling so great that you will also want to embrace Plant Over Processed long-term. You should modify as necessary to fit your needs, your goals, and your lifestyle. You may want to enjoy the occasional processed snack or treat, or a favorite food that includes animal products—it's up to you! You may also want to make exceptions for special occasions or trips out of town—that's totally fine too! Eating raw before dinner may not be realistic for you. If that is the case, modify! This plan is meant to be flexible. The goal is to do what works best for your body and your lifestyle, to eat Plant Over Processed *most* of the time, and to let this be your guiding principle. Knowing how great this way of eating makes you feel will help keep you on track.

stocking your plant-based kitchen

Healthful cooking is easy and fun when you have the right items on hand. On the following pages, I'm going to share my essentials for a plant-based fridge and pantry, many of which you will need for the recipes in the next chapter. When shopping for produce, bulk items and dry goods, and condiments, I recommend buying organic and local ingredients as often as possible. With that said, it's not necessary to revamp your entire kitchen at once, and this may not be realistic depending on your budget. Perhaps it's more doable for you to replace one item in your pantry or fridge with a healthier, organic version each time you go shopping. And as you will see, most of the essential fridge and pantry items that I list below are affordable basics that you can use in a variety of ways.

What I do recommend doing all at once, however, is getting rid of all of those processed foods in your kitchen: cookies, crackers, bags of chips, snack foods, white sugar, white flour, and sugar-laden jams. Look through your pantry and your fridge, and if you find items with listed ingredients that you can't pronounce, get rid of them. That's right, it's a kitchen cleanse! This can be very therapeutic if you allow it. Once your pantry is restocked with healthful options, you will be set up to succeed and it will be much easier for you to make good choices.

Also note: You do not need fancy protein powders and supplements in your pantry to follow this plan. I use a few, which I recommend below and include in a few of the recipes in this book, but they are a personal preference. If I were to recommend just one of these items, it would be a high-quality plant protein powder (which I like to add to smoothies).

Feel free to use these lists as a guide for your own grocery shopping. I recommend

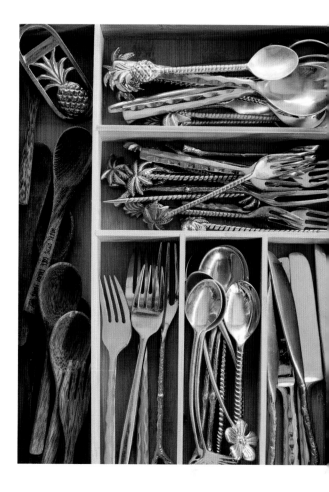

buying items like nuts, seeds, and grains from the bulk aisle whenever possible—it's a great way to save money and use less packaging— and storing them in airtight containers or jars in your pantry. This is what I do in my house, and we also have a few bins in our pantry for miscellaneous items and ingredients like canned goods and healthy snack bars (for convenience!).

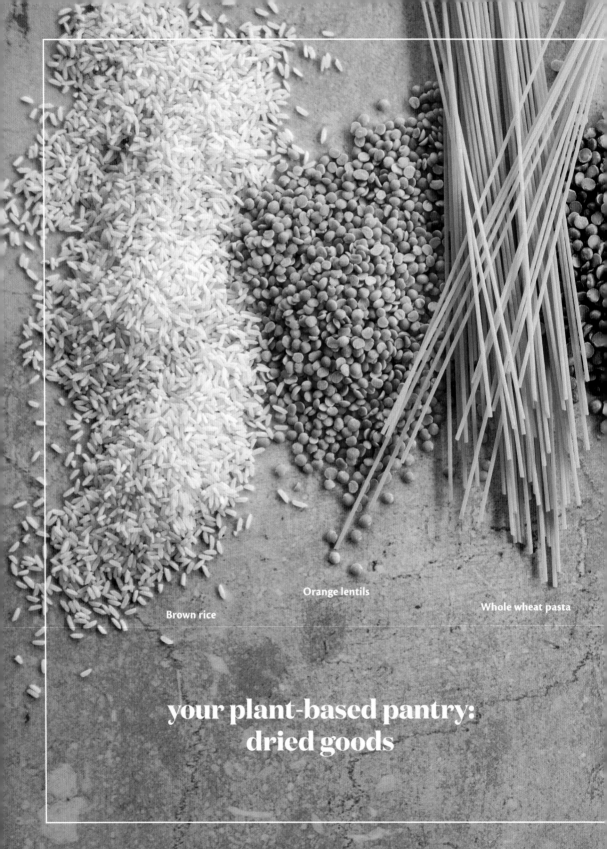

Brown rice

Orange lentils

Whole wheat pasta

your plant-based pantry:
dried goods

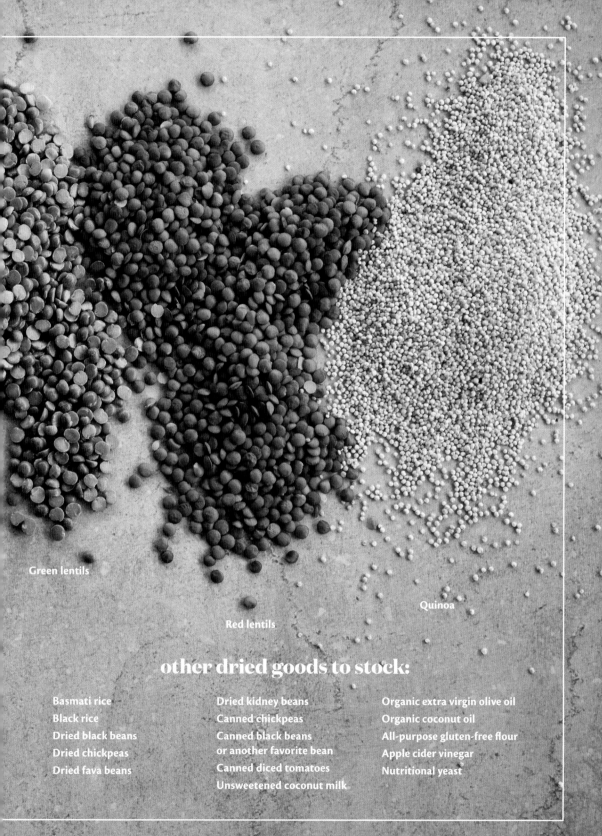

Green lentils

Red lentils

Quinoa

other dried goods to stock:

Basmati rice

Black rice

Dried black beans

Dried chickpeas

Dried fava beans

Dried kidney beans

Canned chickpeas

Canned black beans
or another favorite bean

Canned diced tomatoes

Unsweetened coconut milk

Organic extra virgin olive oil

Organic coconut oil

All-purpose gluten-free flour

Apple cider vinegar

Nutritional yeast

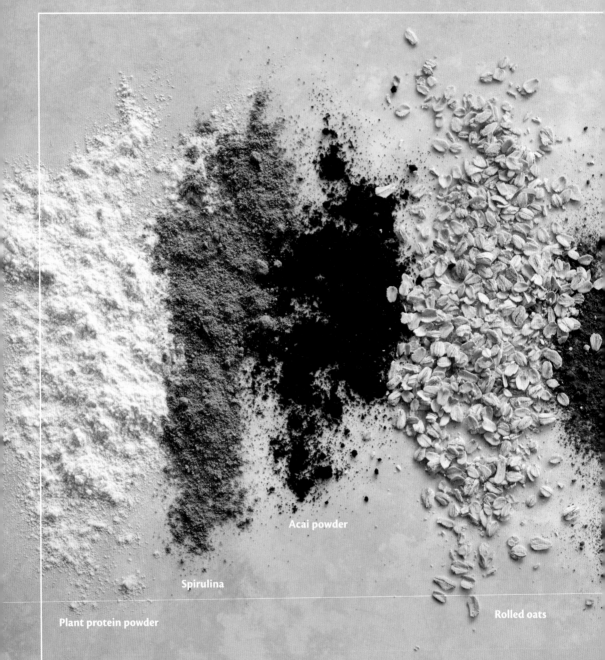

Plant protein powder

Spirulina

Acai powder

Rolled oats

your plant-based pantry:
optional super boosters for smoothies

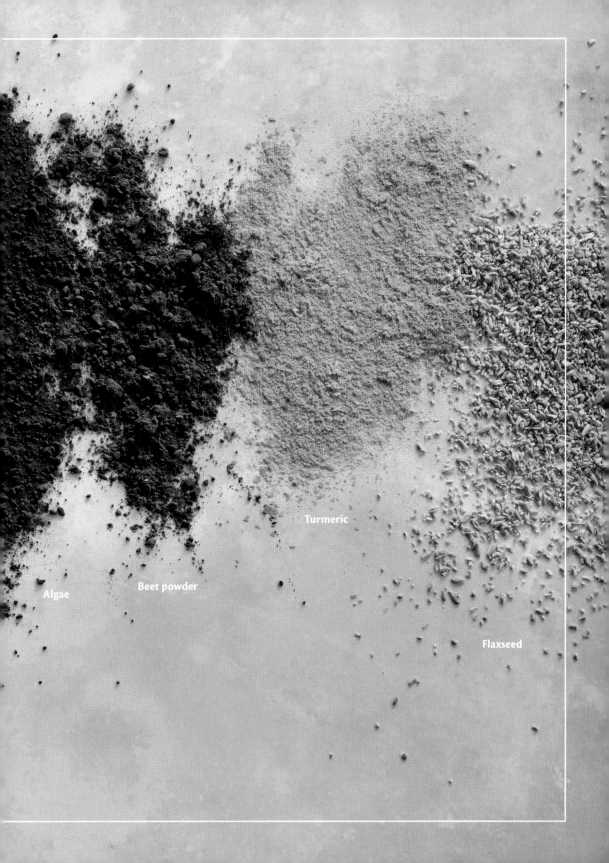

Algae

Beet powder

Turmeric

Flaxseed

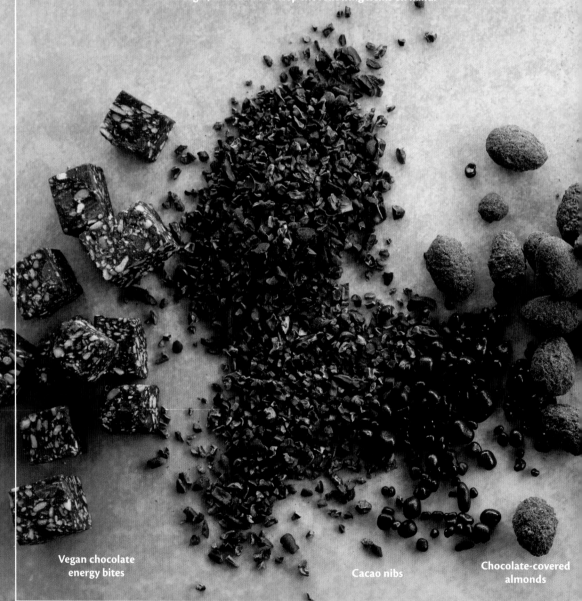

your plant-based pantry: vegan chocolate

When buying vegan chocolate, read ingredient labels and avoid products with food starch and artificial flavorings. Look for higher quality dark chocolate, which is often naturally vegan. Higher quality chocolate is usually made with simple real ingredients such as cacao, cacao butter, little sugar, and vanilla. I keep the following items on hand:

**Vegan chocolate
energy bites**

Cacao nibs

**Chocolate-covered
almonds**

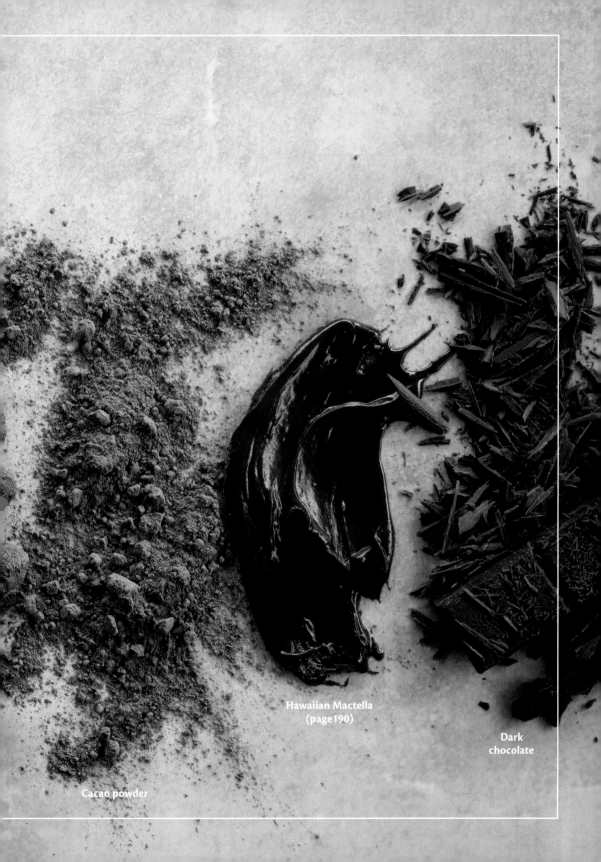

Cacao powder

Hawaiian Mactella
(page190)

Dark
chocolate

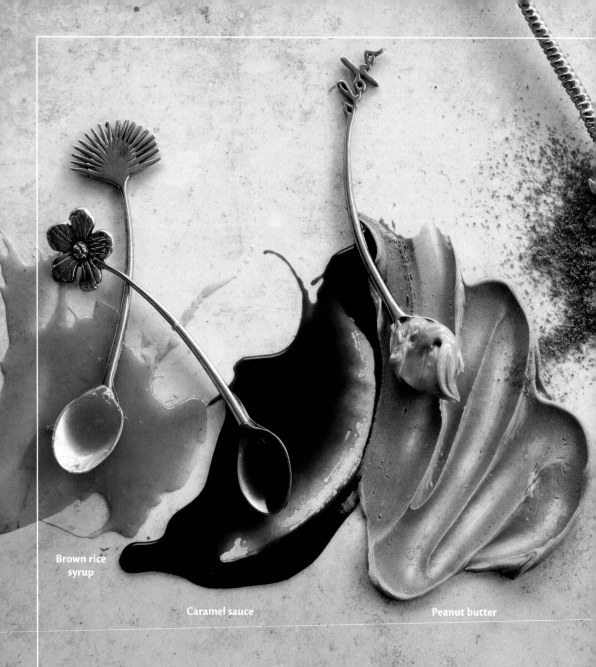

Brown rice
syrup

Caramel sauce

Peanut butter

your plant-based pantry:
sweet toppings and recipe add-ins

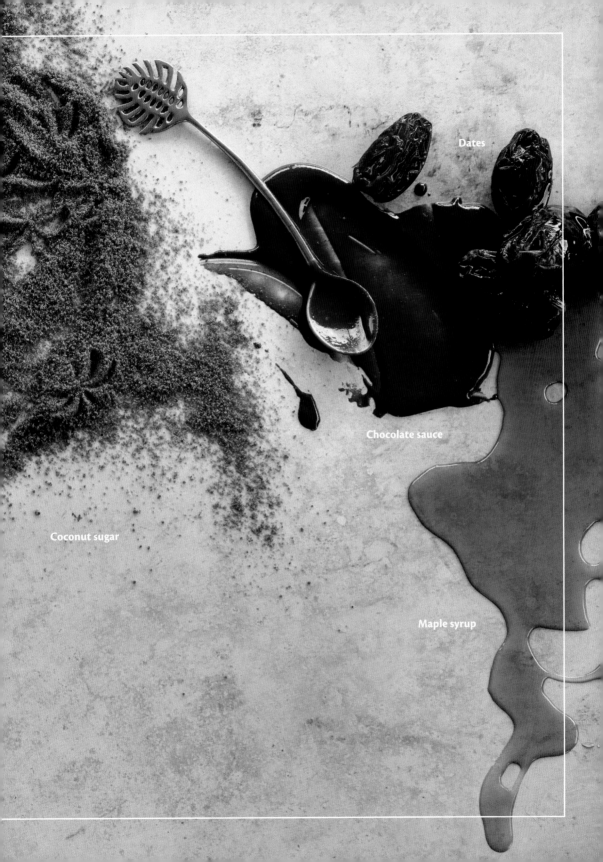

Dates

Chocolate sauce

Coconut sugar

Maple syrup

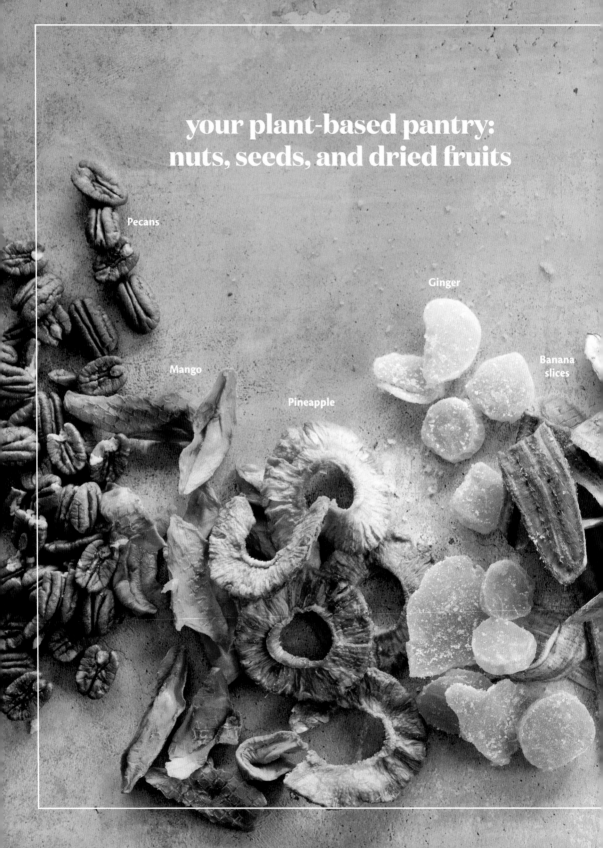

your plant-based pantry: nuts, seeds, and dried fruits

Pecans

Ginger

Mango

Banana slices

Pineapple

other items to stock:

Flaxseeds **Hemp hearts** **Almonds**
Chia seeds **Sunflower seeds** **Pecans**
Pumpkin seeds

Cashews

Banana chips

Mulberries

Coconut

your plant-based pantry: dried spices

Garlic powder

Cumin

Chili flakes

Cinnamon

other items to stock:

Allspice	Chili powder	Oregano
Basil	Cloves	Rosemary
Bay leaves	Dill	Sage
Black peppercorns	Garam masala	Tarragon
Cayenne pepper	Nutmeg	Thyme
	Onion powder	

Curry powder

Seasoning blend

Powdered ginger

Paprika

PLANT-BASED ON A BUDGET

It's a common misconception that eating plant-based must be expensive. I found the opposite—when my family switched to plant-based eating, we began to save money on groceries, as we were no longer purchasing meat and dairy or expensive snack foods, premade dinners, and packaged drinks. Not to mention the money I was saving on doctor's visits and medicines, now that my diet was no longer making me sick!

The real question to ask yourself is whether buying healthy food that costs a bit more is worth the extra money. Is your health, longevity, and quality of life worth the investment? Let me answer this for you: Yes! Spending money on wholesome food is one of the best ways to take care of yourself. And no matter where you live, it is possible to eat plant-based in a way that makes sense for your wallet. Here are some tips for shopping plant-based on a budget:

- **BUY IN BULK:** As mentioned, buying loose items like nuts, seeds, whole grains, and pasta from the bulk aisle in your local grocery store is usually cheaper than buying these items prepackaged. It's also better for the earth too, as you have none of the excess plastic and cardboard packaging, and you can even bring your own reusable cloth bags for these items! You can find all sorts of cloth bags online for just a couple dollars! I prefer organic cotton mesh or cotton muslin for my produce bags. (For more info on ways to reduce packaging, see page 244.)

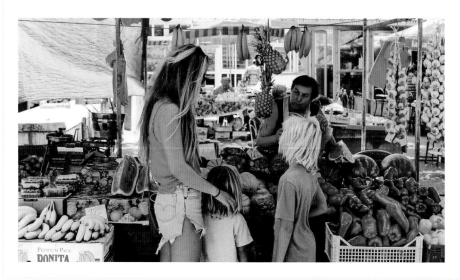

- **BUY IN SEASON:** Foods that are in season tend to be less expensive because they are grown locally rather than flown in or shipped from afar. For the same reason, eating locally lowers your carbon footprint. Foods that are in season usually taste better and are nutritionally superior too.
- **SHOP AT YOUR LOCAL FARMERS MARKET:** Become a regular at your local farmers market, make friends with the vendors there, and look for deals! Once you get to know people and buy from them on a regular basis, they often will be willing to give you special discounts.
- **JOIN A CSA OR BUY A FARM SHARE:** When you join a CSA (Community Supported Agriculture) farm, you are buying a "share" or membership in a local farm, and you typically receive a box of fresh produce each week during the farming season. Some farms even offer discounted memberships in exchange for volunteer work at the farm. Sounds like fun, right? Do some research to see if there is a CSA in your area.
- **CHALLENGE YOURSELF NOT TO WASTE FOOD:** When I first went plant-based, I worried about being able to consume all of the fresh produce I was buying before it went bad! I was nervous about wasting money and food, so I challenged myself to get organized and plan all of my meals at the start of each week, before I went grocery shopping, to cut down on ingredient waste. I encourage you to do the same. Plan out your week of meals *before* you head to the grocery store or the farmers market so you will only buy what you need (with the occasional fun extra) once you get there. This planning can be as simple as deciding that you want to make a big soup and eat a big salad and a smoothie once a day. (For more on reducing food waste, see the following sections.)

stocking your fridge and freezer

I don't keep a lot in my freezer, because I like to know exactly what I have so ingredients don't go to waste. The essentials that are always stocked in my freezer are a variety of frozen fruits for smoothies and bowls, vegetables like avocados or beets that are about to turn and can be used for smoothies, and frozen soups. I always keep the following fruits stocked in my freezer, to use on their own or in combination as a base for my favorite smoothies and smoothie bowls:

Ripe bananas

Mangos (cut into chunks)

Pineapple (cut into chunks)

Blueberries

Acai packets

Strawberries

In my fridge, I like to have leafy greens like kale and spinach on hand to make salads, along with a few fresh herbs for the recipes I plan to make that week, and assorted veggies to be used in meals or as snacks for that week. I also keep a variety of condiments, plant milks, and other miscellaneous items in my fridge. As mentioned, I meal plan at the start of each week and make a list of items that I will need to replenish, depending on the recipes I plan to make for that week. These are the items that I like to keep on hand in my fridge or on the counter at any given time, not necessarily all at once, but depending on the recipes that I plan to make for each week:

VEGETABLES

Spinach

Kale

Cucumbers

Carrots

Potatoes

Sweet potatoes

Broccoli

Cauliflower

Purple cabbage

Green cabbage

Tomatoes

Red onions

White or yellow onions

Garlic

FRESH HERBS

Chives

Cilantro

Mint

Parsley

Basil

CONDIMENTS/SIDES

Mustard (Dijon and stone-ground)

Teriyaki sauce

Coconut aminos or tamari sauce

A favorite hot sauce

Worcestershire sauce (make sure it's vegan)

Pickled ginger (make sure it doesn't contain sugar or coloring)

Sauerkraut

Miso paste

Red curry paste

Capers

Olives

Pickled Red Onions (page 174)

Homemade sauces (made ahead for the week)

PLANT MILKS

When choosing a plant milk, make sure to opt for something that is organic and unsweetened.

Oat milk

Almond milk (or your favorite plant milk)

FRUITS

Whatever fruits are in season, for snacking or to add to smoothie bowls

OTHER

Sourdough bread (which is easier to digest and okay for many who are gluten-intolerant) or gluten-free bread

Corn tortillas

Pita bread (gluten-free)

Tofu

flavor theming—build your own meal plan

Once your 30-Day Plant Over Processed Challenge ends, and you are looking for a sustainable way to stick to this way of eating for life, a great way to stay motivated and stay on track is a little something I call Flavor Theming! Flavor Theming is as much fun as it sounds—it keeps your palate entertained, and it allows you to experiment with a variety of cuisines and travel the globe without leaving your kitchen. It is also incredibly practical, with the added benefits of helping you to meal plan and shop for groceries each week, and to save money, because you will cut down on waste and end up throwing away fewer leftover ingredients.

Flavor theming begins by choosing an area of the world for flavor inspiration at the start of the week and then using that theme as a way of deciding what to cook and narrowing down your search for ingredients at the grocery store that week. My favorite flavor themes, which you will see reflected in the recipes in the next chapter, are Hawaiian (of course), Mexican, Thai, Japanese, and Greek. Before, I might have decided to make a Thai curry on Monday, and then maybe tacos on Tuesday, and spaghetti or burgers on Wednesday, and so on. The problem was that these meals call for a variety of different ingredients, and I always ended up wasting food, or having to run to the store constantly for things I'd run out of or forgotten. Now, each week, I choose one general theme before embarking on my grocery haul, and I find that I am able to reuse and repurpose so many ingredients—fresh herbs, in particular—that would otherwise go to waste.

And if you are thinking, "I don't want to eat *just* Mexican or *just* Thai on any given week," don't worry! Your flavor theme doesn't have to apply to every single dish you eat during a given week. It just serves as a kind of primary guideline for narrowing in on complementary ingredients and then using those ingredients in a variety of ways as the basis of your meals.

Now that you understand the basics of your 30-Day Plant Over Processed Challenge, and you've shopped for groceries and stocked your pantry and fridge, it's time for the fun part: the recipes!

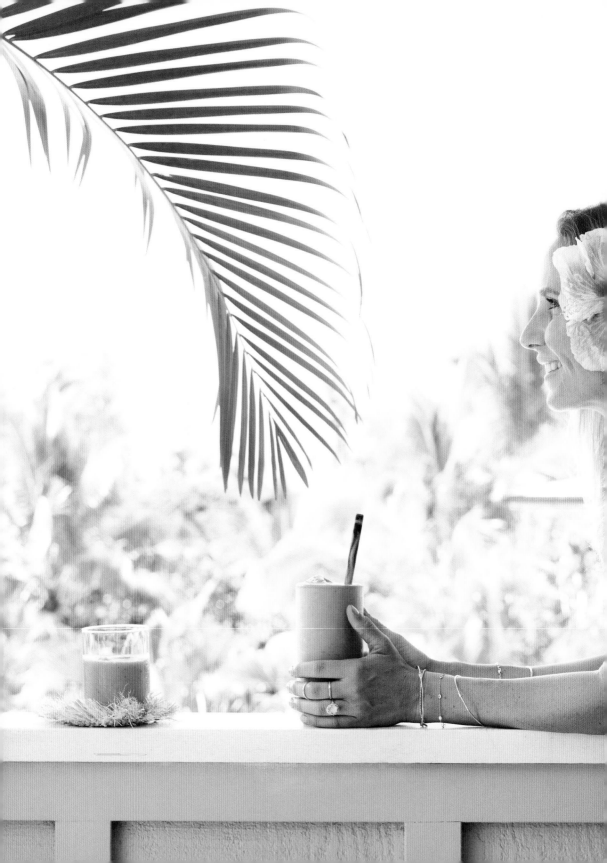

CHAPTER 3

eat the rainbow: plant-based recipes

It's time to eat! In this chapter, we're going to get creative in the kitchen with my favorite plant-based recipes. All of these dishes are easy to make with simple ingredients found at your local grocery store or farmers market. Many of them use the same ingredients in different ways, so that you can make the most out of each of your shopping hauls and reduce food waste. All of these recipes are plant-based and gluten-free, and just as mouthwateringly delicious as they are nutritious! I hope that you will find many favorites here to add to your arsenal.

So here we go! These are my all-time favorite plant-based recipes, developed over the years by cooking with friends, gaining recipe inspiration through travel, and messing around in the kitchen with Shem and the kids. Don't consider yourself a cook? No problem. Success in the kitchen begins with mastering just one or two recipes and building from there. Your ultimate goal is to end up with a regular rotation of yummy, fuss-free recipes in your back pocket that you can whip up on a regular basis for yourself, your family, and your friends. These recipes are the building blocks for a healthy future. Remember that!

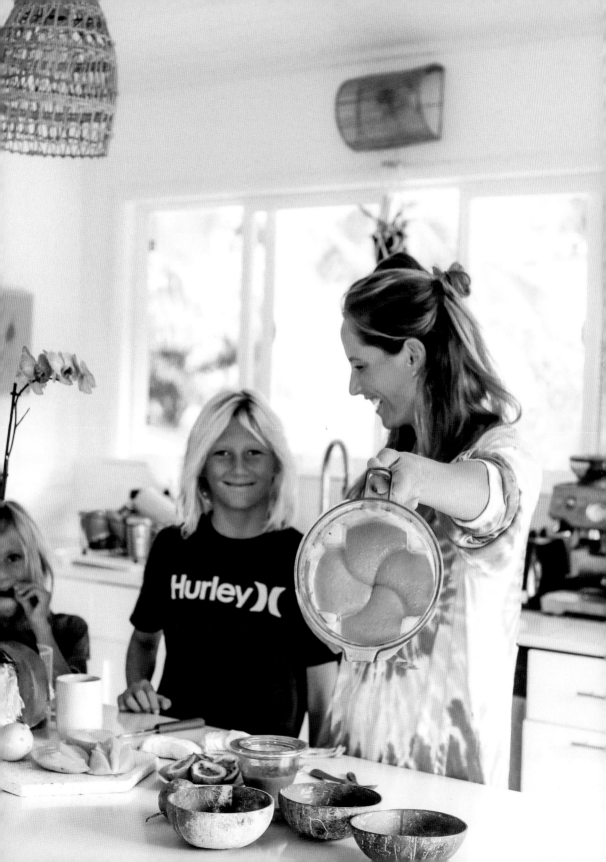

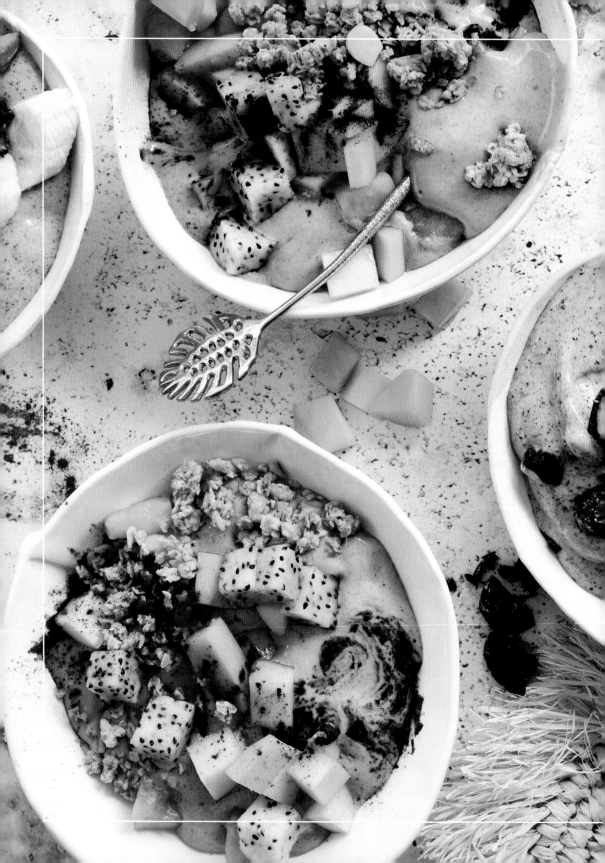

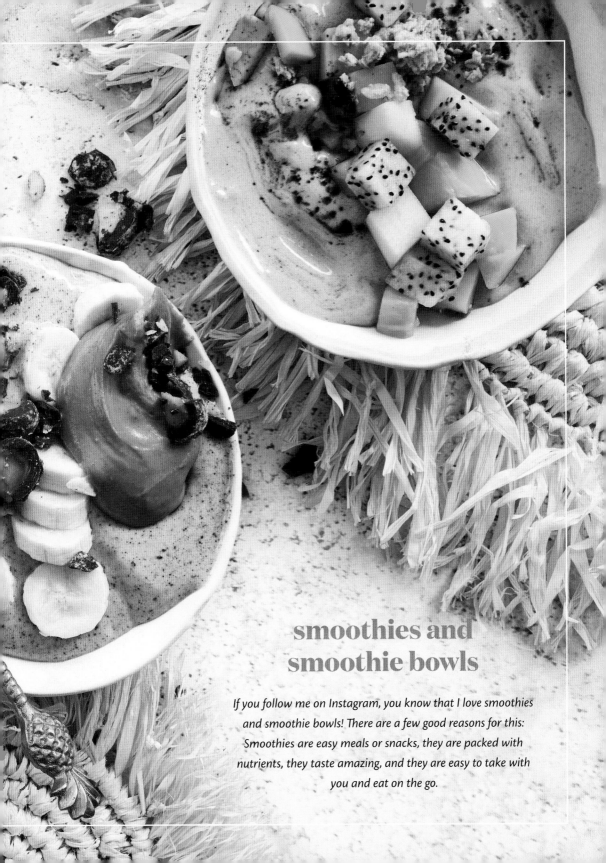

smoothies and smoothie bowls

If you follow me on Instagram, you know that I love smoothies and smoothie bowls! There are a few good reasons for this: Smoothies are easy meals or snacks, they are packed with nutrients, they taste amazing, and they are easy to take with you and eat on the go.

On any given day, I might make a small smoothie for breakfast or a midday snack or a large smoothie for lunch. As a working mom juggling a million things, I often don't get to sit down and enjoy a leisurely meal, and I rely on smoothies and bowls to keep me hydrated and to give me the energy and nutrients I need.

Smoothies and smoothie bowls are also a great vehicle to get my kids to eat whole fruits and vegetables. Because—no surprise—my boys are much more excited about drinking a smoothie than they are about eating a salad! I should note here that they do eat salad a lot, but that was not always the case, so smoothies have been a good way to get in the greens daily! Almost every day after school I make the kids a smoothie. It's easy, quick, nutritious, and satisfying, and the cleanup is breezy.

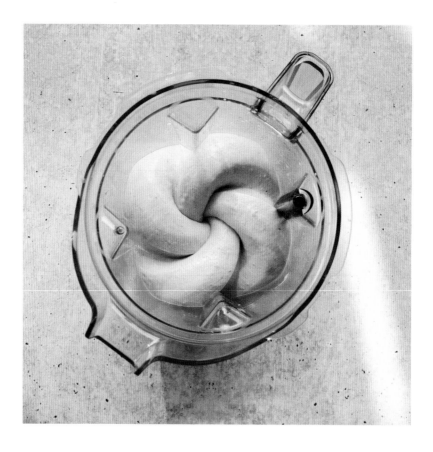

WANT TO BE A SMOOTHIE BOSS?

It's easy! All you have to do is master a few basics. One of the most common questions I'm asked is, "How do you get that thick, creamy texture with your smoothies?" You may be wondering the same thing if your smoothies tend to be on the watery side. Here is your answer, along with my other smoothie secrets:

1. **USE RIPE, SPOTTED FROZEN BANANAS FOR A SWEET AND CREAMY SMOOTHIE BASE.** Ripe bananas give the best flavor and texture and are extremely gentle on the digestive system, whereas unripe bananas can cause bloat and make a smoothie taste like chalk. It makes a world of difference, trust me!

2. **INVEST IN A POWERFUL BLENDER OR FOOD PROCESSOR.** I use a Vitamix blender, which I have had for twelve years! A Vitamix is pricey, but it is the only appliance I use daily. This device is worth every penny as far as I am concerned because it works so well and it will last. Whatever brand you choose, a high-powered blender can be a great health investment. If you are on a budget, look for a secondhand bargain!

3. **USE AS LITTLE LIQUID AS POSSIBLE FOR A THICK SMOOTHIE CONSISTENCY.** The more powerful your blender, the easier it will be to get a thick, creamy consistency because you won't need to add as much liquid. If you don't have access to a powerful blender, you can still make a smoothie; you will just need more liquid in the form of water or your favorite plant milk (mine is oat milk). Your smoothie will still taste great, but the consistency will be thinner. Remember, you can always add liquid, but you can't take it out!

4. **KNOW THE BEST FRUITS TO USE FOR SMOOTHIES VERSUS BOWLS.** For both, I recommend using base fruits that are creamy, such as frozen bananas and mangos. For flavoring and color, I like to add pineapple, blueberries, mangos, tropical fruit mixes, and peaches—these fruits pack a nutritional punch and add amazing color! For smoothie bowls and thicker smoothies, I avoid fruits that are watery, like melons, kiwis, and grapes. These fruits are fine if you don't mind a watery smoothie, however.

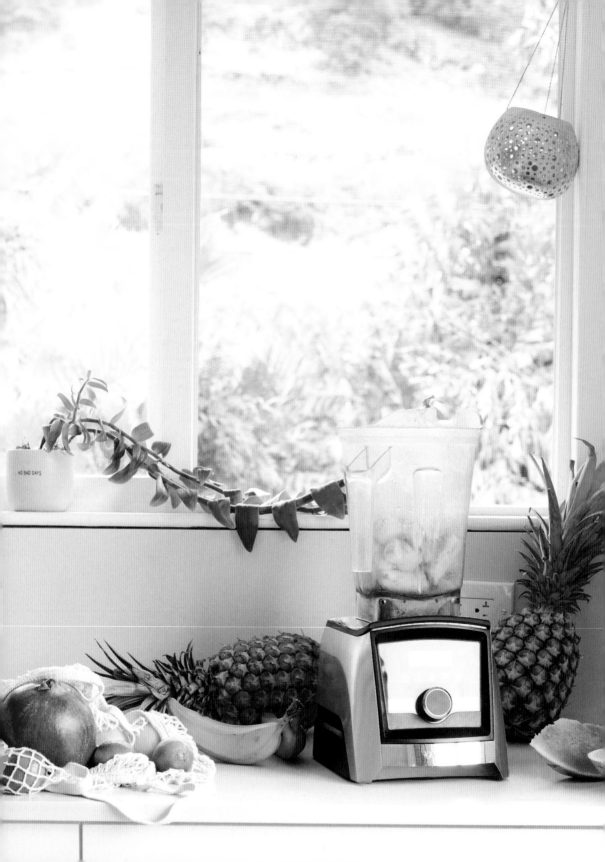

5. **HAVE SUPPLIES ON HAND AND PREPPED IN ADVANCE.** Your prepped smoothie staples should include:

- Frozen fruit and almond milk ice cubes in the freezer. My favorite fruits to freeze for smoothies are bananas, blueberries, mangos, and strawberries, or a tropical fruit mix of pineapple, strawberries, and mango.
- Fresh fruit in the house. Anything that you particularly enjoy and that is in season. My favorite fresh fruits for topping smoothies are blueberries, mangos, and bananas.
- Dry smoothie toppings in jars in the pantry. My favorite dry toppings include shredded coconut, dried fruits, nuts, hemp hearts, granola (see page 97), and dark chocolate or cacao nibs.
- Other favorite smoothie toppings, including nut butters, my homemade vegan Salted Coconut Caramel Sauce (page 196), Andy and Shem's Coconut Yogurt (page 92), or Hawaiian Mactella (page 190).

6. **INCLUDE NUTRIENT-PACKED ADDITIONS TO YOUR SMOOTHIE.** You can add ground flaxseeds, plant protein powder, spirulina, spinach, and kale to any smoothie without altering its taste much.

7. **LOOK OUT FOR THE SWIRL!** Blend your ingredients starting at medium speed and gradually increasing to high while pushing the mixture down with a smoothie wand. You will need to stop the blender periodically to stir the ingredients, repeating until you see that creamy swirl! You might have to stop your blender multiple times within the one to two minutes it takes to reach your end goal. Once you see that swirl, you'll know you've achieved the perfect creamy consistency!

Congratulations, you're a smoothie pro!

TIP: Make your smoothies and bowls even thicker by storing them in the freezer for 30 minutes before you serve! If I am making smoothies for a big group, sometimes I'll blend a whole batch ahead of time and store it in the freezer so that it's ready to go and all of my guests can have nice thick bowls at the same time!

Here are my favorite delicious and nutritious smoothie and smoothie bowl recipes. The difference between a smoothie and a smoothie bowl is pretty simple: a smoothie has a thinner consistency than a smoothie bowl because it contains more liquid, like plant milk or water and a handful of ice. Smoothie bowls contain as little excess liquid as possible, with no added ice, to achieve a thicker consistency. You can make all of the smoothie bowl recipes here into smoothies by adding 1 additional cup of liquid and a handful of ice. Likewise, you can make all of the smoothie recipes into smoothie bowls by eliminating the ice and reducing the amount of liquid you use!

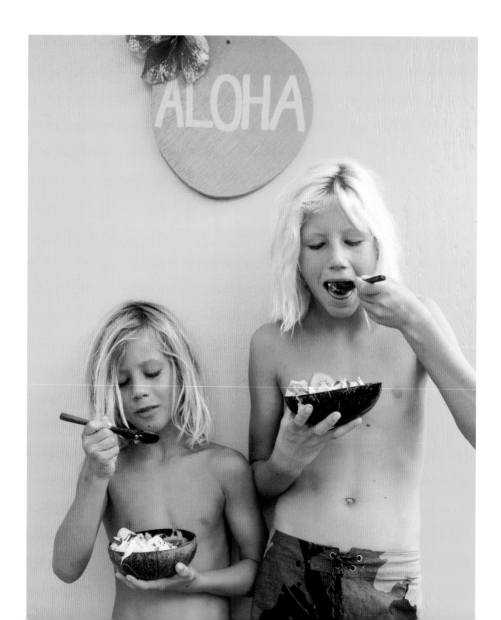

blubana smoothie

PREP TIME: 2 MINUTES • TOTAL TIME: 5 MINUTES • SERVES 2

This is one of my favorite everyday go-to smoothie recipes! The blueberries and bananas are a perfect dancing duo, and I add a little pineapple for a flavorful kick.

2 cups frozen blueberries
2 frozen ripe bananas
1 cup frozen or fresh pineapple chunks (optional)
1 cup ice
1 cup plant milk
1 scoop vanilla protein powder (optional)

1. Place all the ingredients in a high-speed blender.
2. Blend, starting on medium speed and gradually making your way up to high, for 1 to 2 minutes, until the consistency is smooth and creamy. Stop your blender occasionally to mix the ingredients together and push them down with a smoothie stick.

LIVING PLANT-BASED RECIPE

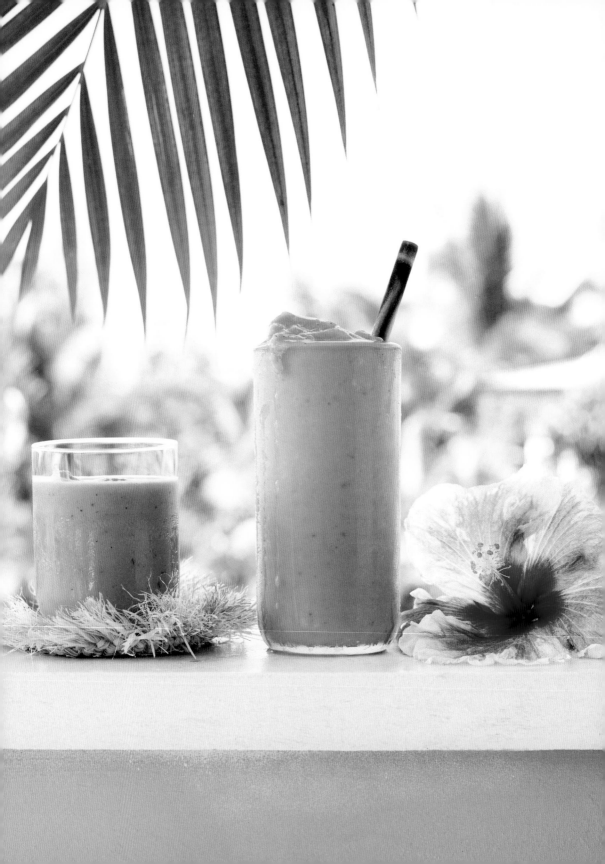

green morning smoothie

PREP TIME: 3 MINUTES • TOTAL TIME: 6 MINUTES • SERVES 2

This is my favorite everyday green smoothie, and my kids love it too! If you are new to the green smoothie world, start here. It tastes super clean and fresh, and it's a great base for adding in other vegetables and fruits, like cucumbers, celery, pears, and peaches.

2 frozen ripe bananas
1 cup spinach or kale leaves
1 cup frozen pineapple or mango chunks
1 cup ice
1 cup plant milk
2 teaspoons vanilla protein powder (optional)
1 teaspoon spirulina or hemp hearts (optional)

1. Place all the ingredients in a high-speed blender.
2. Blend, starting on medium speed and gradually making your way up to high, for 1 to 2 minutes, until the consistency is smooth and creamy. Stop your blender occasionally to mix the ingredients together and push them down with a smoothie stick.

LIVING PLANT-BASED RECIPE

coolin' keiki smoothie

PREP TIME: 3 MINUTES • TOTAL TIME: 5 MINUTES • SERVES 2

This is a smoothie that will make getting your greens super easy! It's so tasty that you won't even realize it's packed with minerals, anti-inflammatory phytonutrients, antioxidants, and fiber.

LIVING PLANT-BASED RECIPE

2 cups spinach or kale leaves
1 heaping cup frozen pineapple or peeled green apple chunks
2 frozen ripe bananas
1 cup plant milk
1 cup ice
¼ cup fresh mint leaves
1 scoop vanilla protein powder (optional)
1 teaspoon spirulina (optional)

1. Place all the ingredients in a high-speed blender.
2. Blend, starting on medium speed and gradually making your way up to high, for 1 to 2 minutes, until the consistency is smooth and creamy. Stop your blender occasionally to mix the ingredients together and push them down with a smoothie stick.

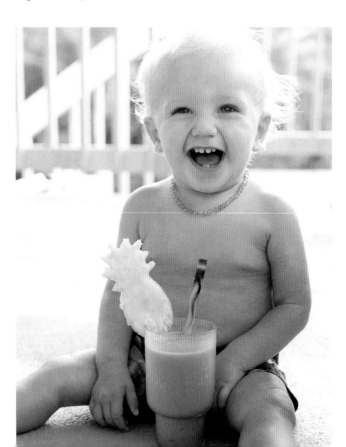

chai chai shake

PREP TIME: 4 MINUTES • TOTAL TIME: 6 MINUTES • SERVES 2

A healthy, nutrient-packed chocolate chai milkshake? Is such a thing even possible? Yes! Prepare to indulge, knowing that this decadent shake is actually good for you!

1½ cups plant milk
3 frozen ripe bananas
1 tablespoon cacao powder
½ teaspoon ground cinnamon
⅛ teaspoon ground nutmeg
½ teaspoon pure vanilla extract
⅛ teaspoon ground cloves
⅛ teaspoon ground cardamom
¼ teaspoon ground ginger
1 piece crystallized ginger or 1 teaspoon grated ginger (optional, but next level)
4 pitted Medjool dates or 1 tablespoon maple syrup
1 cup ice

1. Place all the ingredients in a high-speed blender.
2. Blend, starting on medium speed and gradually making your way up to high, for 1 to 2 minutes, until the consistency is smooth and creamy. Stop your blender occasionally to mix the ingredients together and push them down with a smoothie stick.

LIVING PLANT-BASED RECIPE

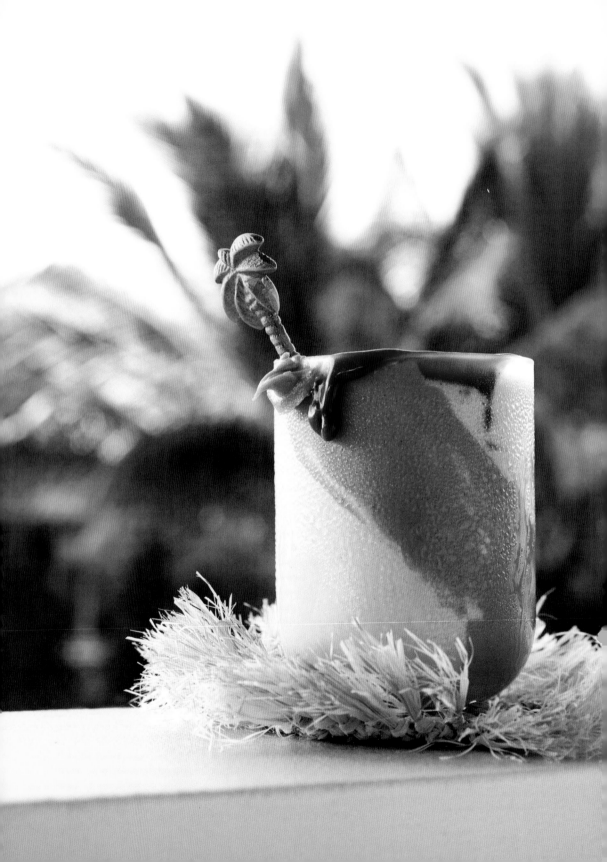

peanut butter paradise smoothie

PREP TIME: 2 MINUTES • TOTAL TIME: 4 MINUTES • SERVES 2

We should really be calling this smoothie Fifty Shades of Peanut Butter. If you're a peanut butter lover, you will be all over this thick shake!

¼ cup natural peanut butter
4 frozen ripe bananas
1 cup plant milk
¼ cup vanilla protein powder (optional)
2 to 3 pitted Medjool dates or 2 teaspoons coconut sugar (optional, but yummy!)
1 cup ice

1. Place all the ingredients in a high-speed blender.
2. Blend, starting on medium speed and gradually making your way up to high, for 1 to 2 minutes, until the consistency is smooth and creamy. Stop your blender occasionally to mix the ingredients together and push them down with a smoothie stick.

LIVING PLANT-BASED RECIPE

apple pie shake

PREP TIME: 5 MINUTES • TOTAL TIME: 7 MINUTES • SERVES 2

If you want apple pie, have apple pie! This smoothie tastes like a holiday dessert, but it will hydrate you and do your body good with loads of vitamins, fiber, and minerals!

1 cup plant milk
1 tablespoon vanilla protein powder (optional)
¼ cup gluten-free rolled oats
1 medium apple, peeled, cored, and chopped
1 frozen ripe banana
½ teaspoon pure vanilla extract
1 teaspoon maple syrup or 2 pitted Medjool dates
1 teaspoon pumpkin pie spice
1 cup ice

1. Place all the ingredients in a high-speed blender.

2. Blend, starting on medium speed and gradually making your way up to high, for 1 to 2 minutes, until the consistency is smooth and creamy. Stop your blender occasionally to mix the ingredients together and push them down with a smoothie stick.

LIVING PLANT-BASED RECIPE

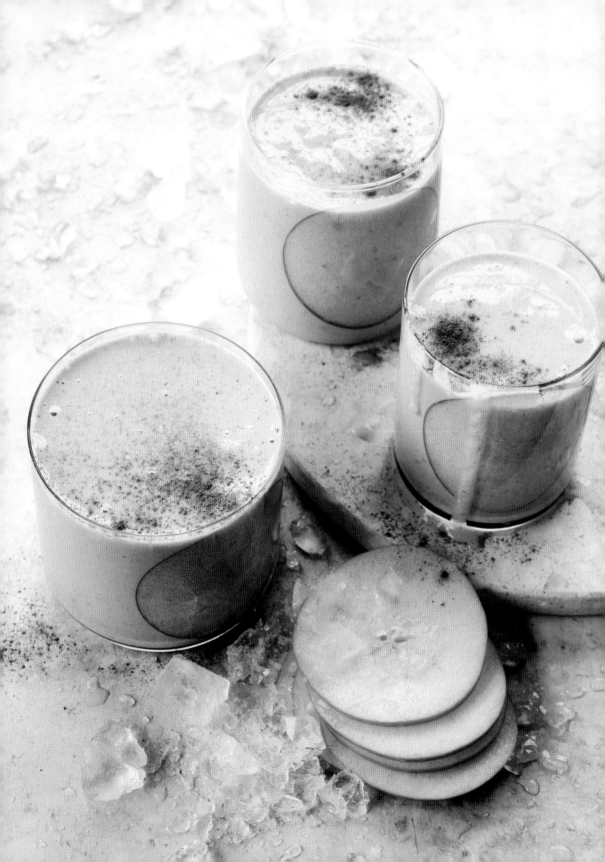

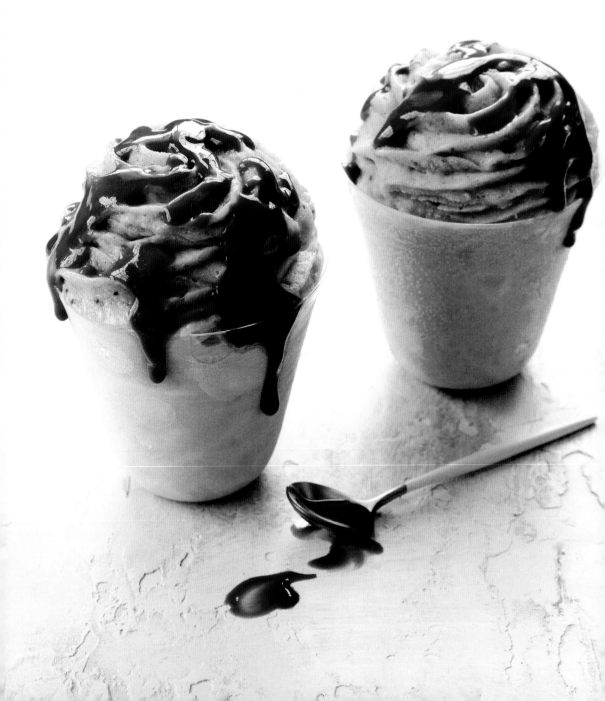

salted caramel banilla smoothie

PREP TIME: 3 MINUTES • TOTAL TIME: 5 MINUTES • SERVES 2

I die for salted caramel, so I came up with a way to have it every day and still be healthy. This smoothie tastes naughty but is a whole lot of nice packed with minerals, protein, vitamins, and fiber to keep you feeling your best!

2 frozen ripe bananas
2 to 3 pitted Medjool dates or 1 tablespoon coconut sugar
½ teaspoon pure vanilla extract
1 cup plant milk
1 cup ice
1 tablespoon vanilla protein powder (optional)
Salted Coconut Caramel Sauce (page 192) for topping

1. Place all the ingredients except the salted coconut caramel sauce in a high-speed blender.

2. Blend, starting on medium speed and gradually making your way up to high, for 1 to 2 minutes, until the consistency is smooth and creamy. Stop your blender occasionally to mix the ingredients together and push them down with a smoothie stick.

3. Drizzle with the salted coconut caramel sauce.

LIVING PLANT-BASED RECIPE

frozen hot chocolate smoothie

PREP TIME: 3 MINUTES • TOTAL TIME: 5 MINUTES • SERVES 2

This is the perfect chocolate shake, only it's made from healthy ingredients that will keep you feeling your best! This is one I love to make for breakfast or as an afternoon snack when the sweet tooth strikes.

2 to 3 frozen ripe bananas
2 to 3 pitted Medjool dates or 1 tablespoon coconut sugar
½ teaspoon pure vanilla extract
1 cup plant milk
1 cup ice
1 tablespoon vanilla or chocolate plant protein powder (optional)
1 tablespoon cacao powder

1. Place all the ingredients in a high-speed blender.
2. Blend, starting on medium speed and gradually making your way up to high, for 1 to 2 minutes, until the consistency is smooth and creamy. Stop your blender occasionally to mix the ingredients together and push them down with a smoothie stick.

LIVING PLANT-BASED RECIPE

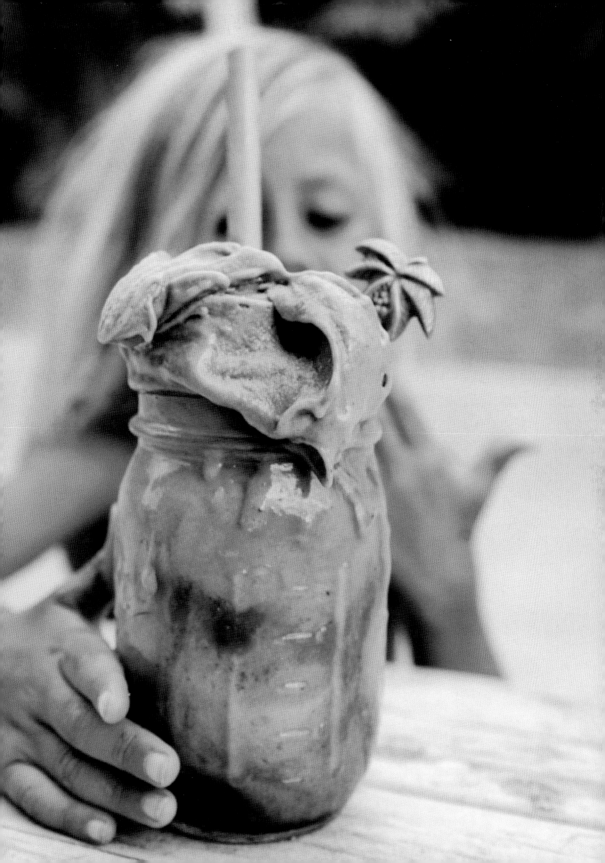

INSTAGRAM-WORTHY SMOOTHIE BOWLS

It's easier than you think to make gorgeous and delicious smoothie bowls. First, follow my Smoothie Boss instructions (see pages 65–67) for getting that perfect thick, creamy texture, and then once your bowl is poured, decorate it with your favorite scrumptious toppings. The key to making your bowl pretty and photo-op ready is arranging your toppings in flowy "moon" shapes. I like to top my bowls with a dollop of nut butter, sliced banana, and granola. And when I want something a bit chewy, for texture I'll also add goji berries, dried blueberries, finely diced dried mango, or mochi. Feel free to get as wild or as simple with your toppings as you like!

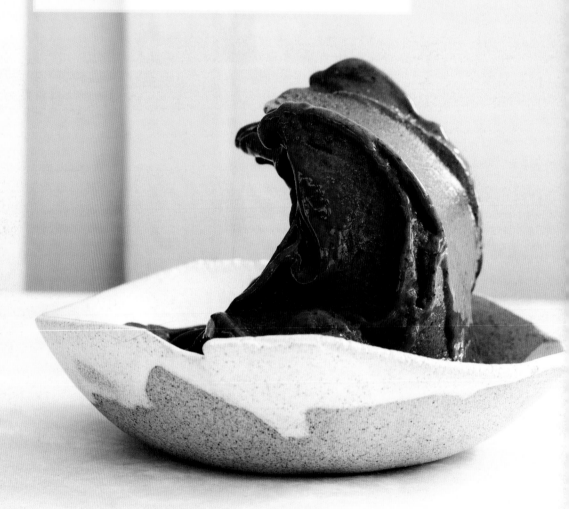

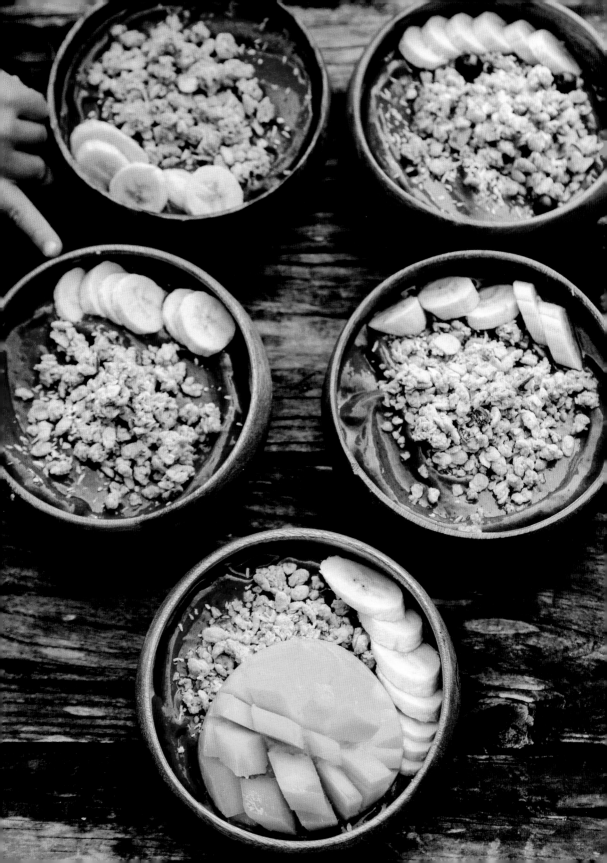

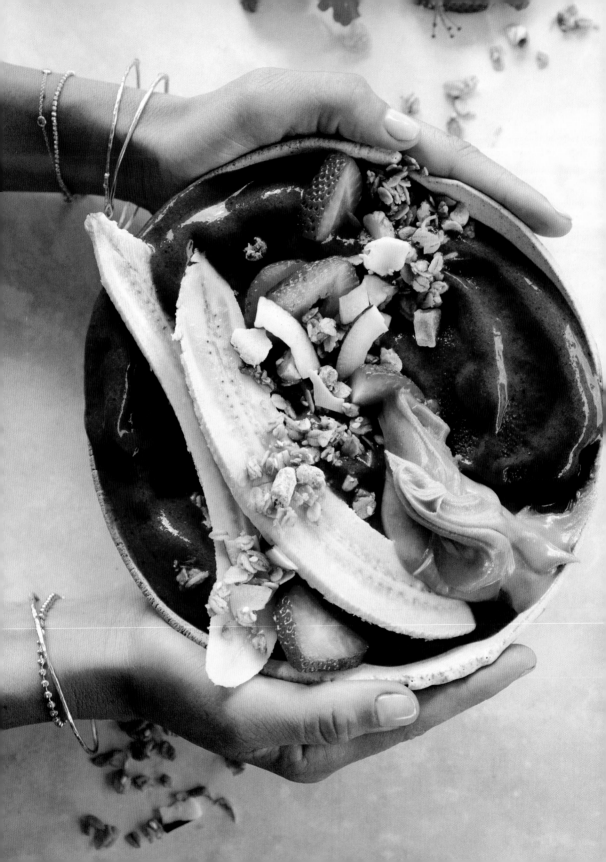

og acai bowl

PREP TIME: 5 MINUTES • TOTAL TIME: 8 MINUTES • SERVES 1 TO 2

Barely a day goes by when our blender isn't whipping up an acai bowl. There is something addictive about acai bowls, and as far as addictions go, this is a good one! Get hooked on the antioxidant- and vitamin-rich sweetness of this fruity acai bowl with all the trimmings!

2 cups frozen blueberries
3 frozen ripe bananas
2 (3.5-ounce) acai superfruit packs or 1 scoop acai powder
1 cup frozen mango chunks
½ cup plant milk
Toppings: sliced banana, granola, shredded coconut, goji berries, mango, blueberries, kiwi

1. Place all the ingredients except the toppings in a high-powered blender.

2. Blend, starting on medium speed and gradually making your way up to high, for 1 to 2 minutes, stopping every 20 seconds or so to mix the ingredients and push them down with a smoothie stick. Once you see the "swirl," you will know it's done.

3. Pour your smoothie into your favorite bowl and add your choice of toppings.

LIVING PLANT-BASED RECIPE

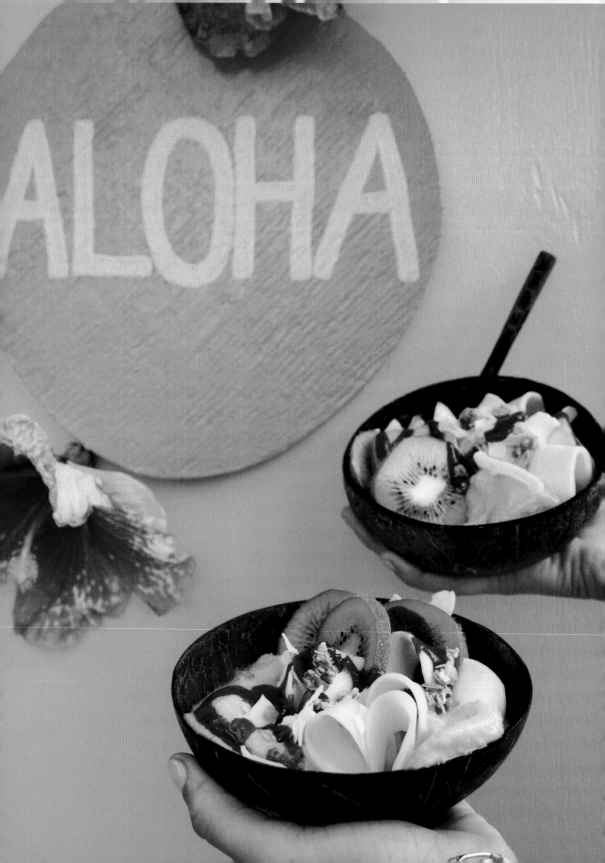

sunrise shack bowl

PREP TIME: 5 MINUTES • TOTAL TIME: 8 MINUTES • SERVES 1 TO 2

This bowl is inspired by a little snack shack down the street from us called the Sunrise Shack that is run by the nicest group of guys you'll ever meet! They are always spreading good vibes with their healthy treats, which is why I named this bowl after them. There's an anti-inflammatory health boost in every hydrating bite.

1 cup frozen mango chunks
2 frozen ripe bananas
½ cup frozen or fresh pineapple chunks
1 teaspoon ground turmeric
¼ cup plant milk
Toppings: sliced banana, dragon fruit, mango, granola, shredded coconut

1. Place all the ingredients except the toppings in a high-powered blender.

2. Blend, starting on medium speed and gradually making your way up to high, for 1 to 2 minutes, stopping every 20 seconds or so to mix the ingredients and push them down with a smoothie stick. Once you see the "swirl," you will know it's done.

3. Pour your smoothie into your favorite bowl and add your choice of toppings.

LIVING PLANT-BASED RECIPE

blue room bowl

PREP TIME: 3 MINUTES • TOTAL TIME: 6 MINUTES • SERVES 1 TO 2

In surfer speak, the view from inside the barrel of a wave is called the "blue room." For those of us who can't get barreled, but who still want to hang out in the blue room, there is this delicious, tropical smoothie bowl! Blue-green algae and spirulina, both of which can be found in most health food stores, are full of powerful antioxidants and anti-inflammatory properties. And they are what gives this bowl its color!

2 cups frozen tropical fruit mix (papaya, pineapple, mango, strawberries)
2 frozen ripe bananas
½ cup plant milk
1 teaspoon blue-green algae or spirulina
Toppings: sliced banana, dragon fruit, diced mango, granola, coconut shreds

1. Place all the ingredients except the toppings in a high-powered blender.
2. Blend, starting on medium speed and gradually making your way up to high, for 1 to 2 minutes, stopping every 20 seconds or so to mix the ingredients and push them down with a smoothie stick. Once you see the "swirl," you will know it's done.
3. Pour your smoothie into your favorite bowl and add your choice of toppings.

LIVING PLANT-BASED RECIPE

chunky monkey bowl

PREP TIME: 6 MINUTES • TOTAL TIME: 10 MINUTES • SERVES 1 TO 2

The Chunky Monkey Bowl tastes like a dessert, but it is healthy enough to have for breakfast, which is why it's my kids' favorite. I came up with this recipe for an event we did during the Billabong Pipe Masters surf contest years ago. We created a smoothie bowl truck and handed out eight hundred free smoothie bowls to those in attendance. Good times!

LIVING PLANT-BASED RECIPE

2 to 3 frozen ripe bananas
¼ cup natural peanut or almond butter
¼ cup almond milk (or any nut milk)
¼ cup chocolate protein powder or cacao powder
Toppings: sliced banana, granola, vegan chocolate chips, shredded coconut, and a slab of peanut butter!

1. Place all the ingredients except the toppings in a high-powered blender.
2. Blend, starting on medium speed and gradually making your way up to high, for 1 to 2 minutes, stopping every 20 seconds or so to mix the ingredients and push them down with a smoothie stick. Once you see the "swirl," you will know it's done.
3. Pour your smoothie into your favorite bowl and add your choice of toppings.

DIY MASON JAR TOPPINGS BAR FOR SMOOTHIE BOWLS

In our house, we *always* keep the pantry stocked with everything we need to create a smoothie bowl smorgasbord! To create a smoothie bowl toppings bar in your home, buy six to ten mason jars and fill each one with your favorite smoothie bowl toppings, to keep in your pantry and have at the ready. This way, your toppings are ready to go whenever you crave a delicious bowl for breakfast or a snack. These same dry toppings can also be combined to make trail mix, or used as yummy add-ins for your homemade granola (see page 97).

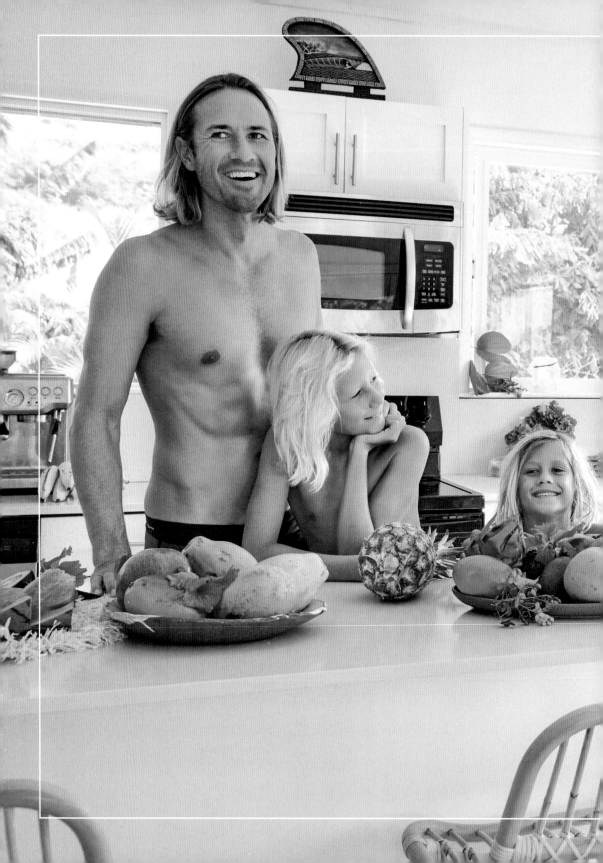

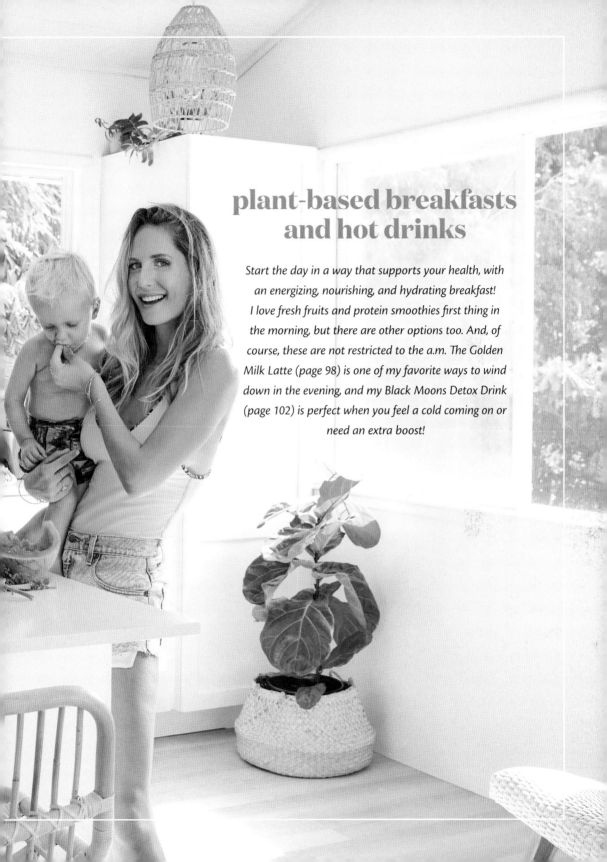

plant-based breakfasts and hot drinks

Start the day in a way that supports your health, with an energizing, nourishing, and hydrating breakfast! I love fresh fruits and protein smoothies first thing in the morning, but there are other options too. And, of course, these are not restricted to the a.m. The Golden Milk Latte (page 98) is one of my favorite ways to wind down in the evening, and my Black Moons Detox Drink (page 102) is perfect when you feel a cold coming on or need an extra boost!

andy and shem's coconut yogurt

PREP TIME: 5 MINUTES • TOTAL TIME: 20 MINUTES + 2 DAYS • SERVES 2

One day Shem and I performed a yogurt experiment. We bought every kind of vegan yogurt at our local Whole Foods, tasted all of them, and, $100 later and disappointed, we decided to make our own! This is a delicious recipe for homemade vegan yogurt that will also save you some cash. The store-bought stuff can be pricey!

You can find the probiotics called for in this recipe in most health food stores. The 50 billion live cultures make all the difference.

LIVING PLANT-BASED RECIPE

1 (14-ounce) can full-fat unsweetened coconut milk
2 capsules probiotic with 50 billion live cultures
1 vanilla bean or 1 teaspoon vanilla paste (optional)

EQUIPMENT:
Mason jar
Cheesecloth
Rubber band or string

1. Shake up the can of coconut milk to mix before opening. Pour the coconut milk into a mason jar.

2. Empty the contents of the probiotic capsules into your coconut milk and discard the capsule shells. Stir the probiotic into the milk until it has completely dissolved.

3. If using, cut the vanilla bean lengthwise down the center and use a spoon to scrape the seeds from one half of the bean into your coconut milk. (Save the other half for another recipe.)

4. Cover the top of the mason jar with a single layer of cheesecloth, secure it with a rubber band or string, and leave on your kitchen counter for 24 hours.

5. The top layer should have a thick and airy texture. Stir the yogurt for 10 to 15 seconds, secure the cheesecloth back on the jar, and let sit for an additional 24 hours.

6. After allowing your yogurt to sit for a full 48 hours, remove the cheesecloth and again mix in the thick and creamy top layer with the rest. Cover your mason jar with a lid and place in the fridge to thicken up and chill for an additional 4 to 6 hours.

7. Enjoy your yogurt with your favorite toppings. Add a sweetener like agave syrup or coconut sugar if you like. Yogurt is a waiting game, but it's worth it!

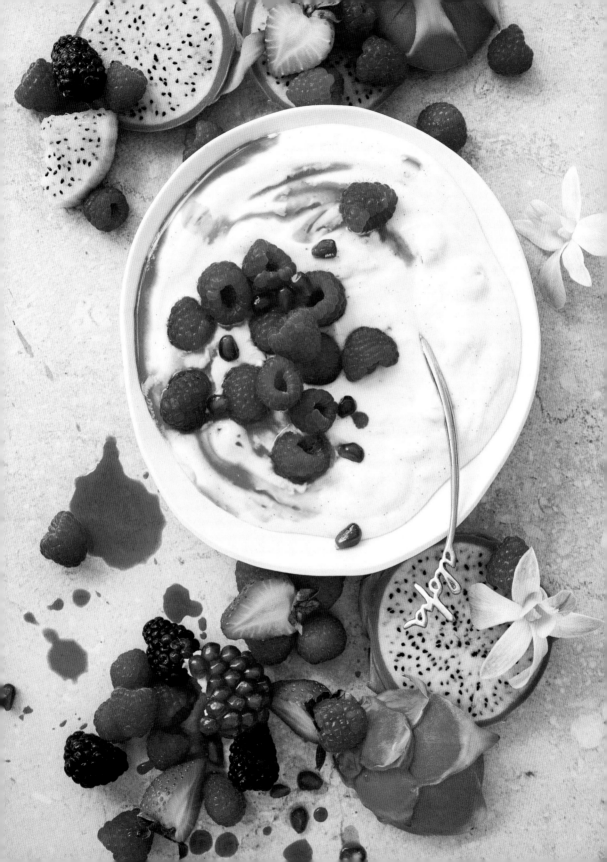

digestion-boosting morning tonic

PREP TIME: 2 MINUTES • TOTAL TIME: 2 MINUTES • SERVES 1

When I first started hanging out with Shem, I came down with the flu and he nursed me back to health with this drink, along with a foot rub. How could I not fall in love? Today we make this drink for our kids whenever one of them gets a cold or needs an extra healing boost. I love this drink because it's made with love!

1 cup filtered water
2 tablespoons fresh lemon juice
⅛ teaspoon cayenne pepper
1 teaspoon maple syrup

1. Whisk all the ingredients together in a small saucepan and heat over medium heat until simmering, 2 to 3 minutes.
2. Pour into a mug and drink hot, while wrapped in a blanket!

LIVING PLANT-BASED RECIPE

citrus splashed fruit

PREP TIME: 4 MINUTES • TOTAL TIME: 4 MINUTES • SERVES: 1

Start your day with fresh fruit! This is one of my favorite breakfast dishes, as I find that fresh fruit is one of the gentlest things on an empty stomach in the morning and great for digestion. That lime-y tang complements all fruits so well!

LIVING PLANT-BASED RECIPE

1 papaya
1 lime
2 whole lilikoi, yellow passion fruit from Hawaii (optional)

Slice a papaya in half. Remove the papaya seeds with a spoon. Now slice your lime and lilikoi if you are using it and squeeze over the papaya flesh. You can eat the seeds of a lilikoi in case you didn't know! Eat immediately!

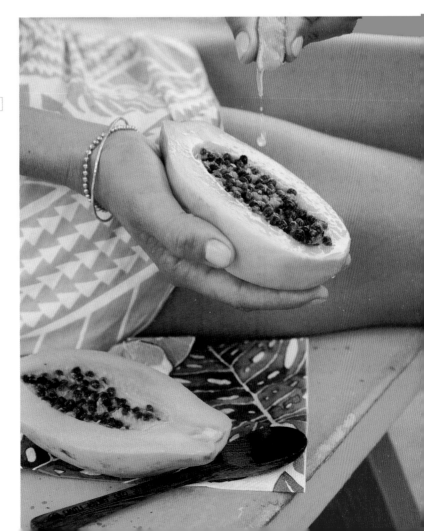

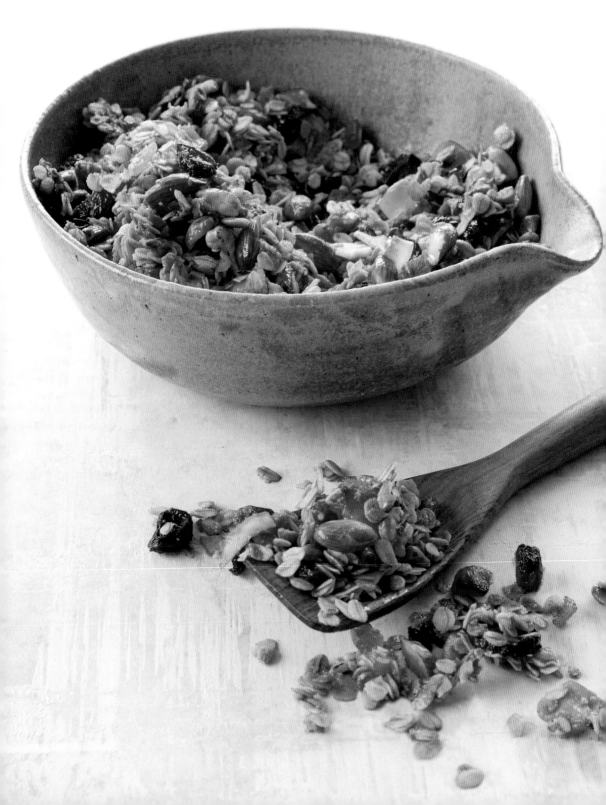

og earthy granola

PREP TIME: 15 MINUTES • TOTAL TIME: 50 MINUTES • SERVES 10

Store-bought granola often contains extra sugars and additives that you don't want, so why not make your own? Not only is it healthier, but it's easy to do and half the price. You can add whatever you like to make it your own, and it will make your kitchen smell like heaven as it's baking!

⅓ cup maple syrup
⅓ cup packed coconut sugar
4 teaspoons pure vanilla extract
½ teaspoon sea salt
½ cup coconut oil, melted
5 cups old-fashioned gluten-free rolled oats
2 cups raw almonds or pistachios, coarsely chopped
2 cups mixed dried fruit of your choice, such as dried blueberries, cherries, mango, and shredded coconut

1. Adjust an oven rack to the upper-middle position and preheat the oven to 325°F. Line a baking sheet with parchment paper.

2. In a large bowl, whisk together the maple syrup, coconut sugar, vanilla, and salt. Then whisk in the coconut oil. Fold in the oats and almonds until thoroughly coated.

3. Transfer the oat mixture to the lined baking sheet and spread across in an even layer. Using a stiff metal spatula, compress the oat mixture until very compact.

4. Bake until lightly browned, 30 to 35 minutes, rotating the pan once halfway through baking. Remove the granola from the oven, spoon into a bowl, and stir in the dried fruit. Allow the mixture to cool before breaking the granola into pieces.

5. Store the granola in a glass jar on the counter for up to 1 month.

COOKED PLANT-BASED RECIPE

golden milk latte

PREP TIME: 3 MINUTES • TOTAL TIME: 10 MINUTES • SERVES: 2

I love bedtime snacks, and before I went Plant Over Processed you could find me eating a bowl of cereal or a pan of Rice Krispie squares before bed. But do you know what? I never woke up feeling great. Now my go-to bedtime snack is a warm, cozy Golden Milk Latte. It smells delicious, warms my belly, and its anti-inflammatory properties help me to wake up feeling fresh.

1½ cups oat milk (or your favorite plant milk)
1 teaspoon grated fresh turmeric or ½ teaspoon ground turmeric
1 teaspoon grated fresh ginger or ¼ teaspoon ground ginger
1½ teaspoons coconut sugar or maple syrup, or 1 pitted Medjool date, finely chopped
¼ teaspoon ground cinnamon, plus extra for garnish

1. Whisk all the ingredients together in a small saucepan and heat over medium heat, 4 to 5 minutes. Once heated, pour into mugs.
2. Sprinkle with additional cinnamon and serve immediately.

PREDOMINANTLY LIVING PLANT-BASED RECIPE

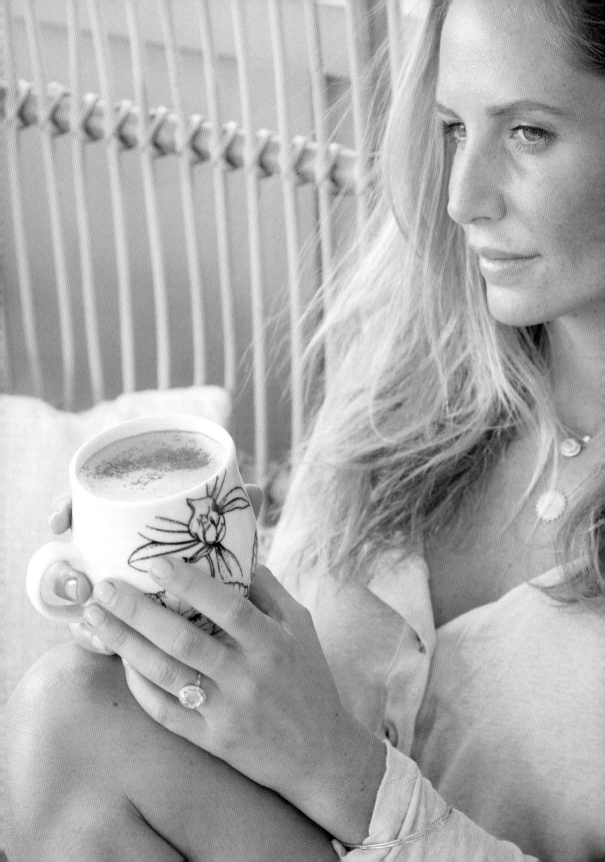

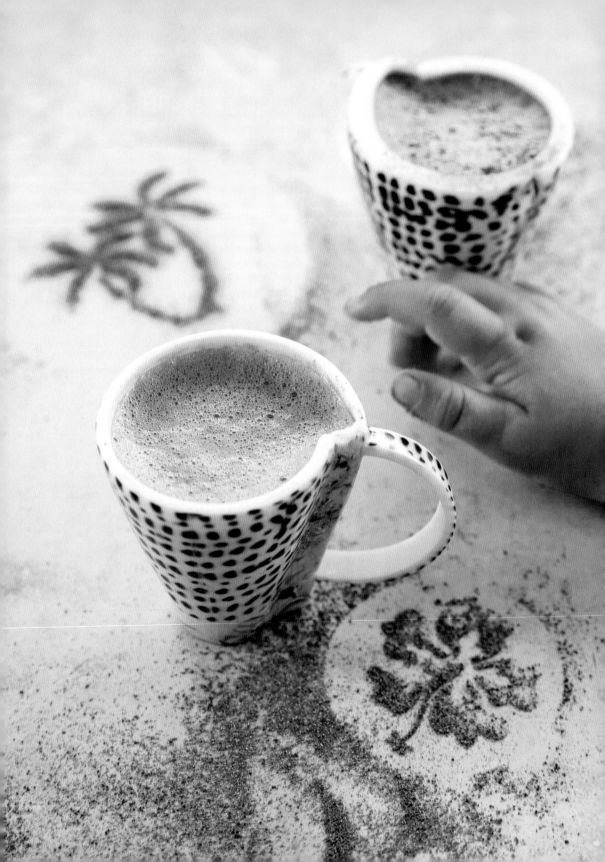

babyccino

PREP TIME: 6 MINUTES • TOTAL TIME: 8 MINUTES • SERVES 1

We had our first "babyccino" with the kids on a sailing trip through Croatia with our Slovenian friends. The kids still ask for it, so we re-created this delicious drink at home— it's the perfect swap for sugary hot chocolate. Combine a little steamed oat or almond milk with a sprinkle of cacao powder and you've got yourself a European-inspired delicacy!

1 cup oat or almond milk
1 teaspoon coconut sugar
1 tablespoon cacao powder, plus extra for topping

1. Whisk all the ingredients together in a saucepan and heat over medium heat, 2 to 3 minutes. Pour into a mug.
2. Sprinkle with a little extra cacao powder and serve.

PREDOMINANTLY LIVING PLANT-BASED RECIPE

black moons detox drink

PREP TIME: 2 MINUTES • TOTAL TIME: 3 MINUTES • SERVES 1

This drink contains activated charcoal, which acts like a sponge to soak up impurities in the body. Black Moons cleanses your system, boosts your energy, aids digestion, and beats bloat. Some even claim that this drink will cure a hangover! Generally speaking, it assists with healing processes in the body. I like to drink this if I'm under the weather or to prevent getting sick while traveling.

1 tablespoon fresh lemon juice
½ teaspoon activated charcoal
1 teaspoon maple syrup
Tiny pinch Himalayan salt
1 cup filtered water
Crushed ice for serving

1. Combine all the ingredients in a jug or pitcher, then pour into a 16-ounce glass over crushed ice.
2. Drink and wait for the energizing, detoxifying results!

LIVING PLANT-BASED RECIPE

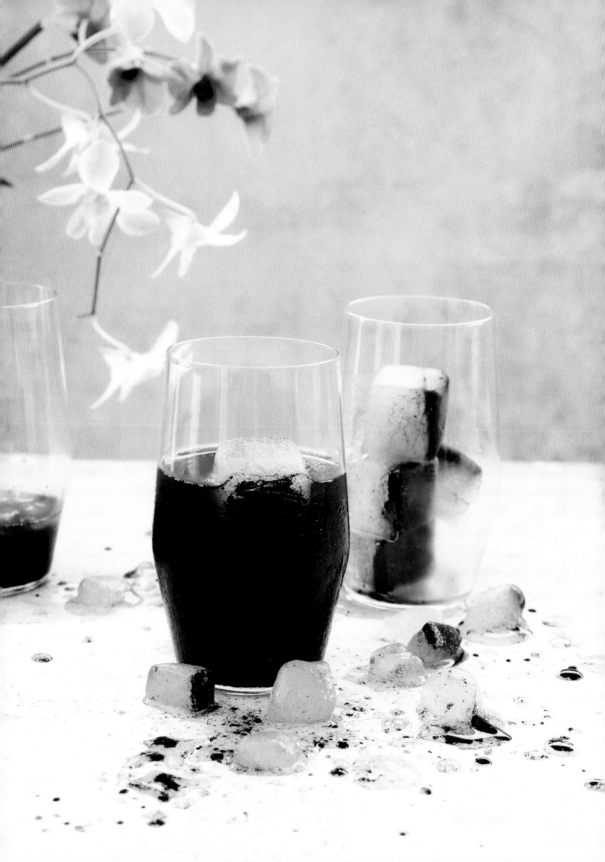

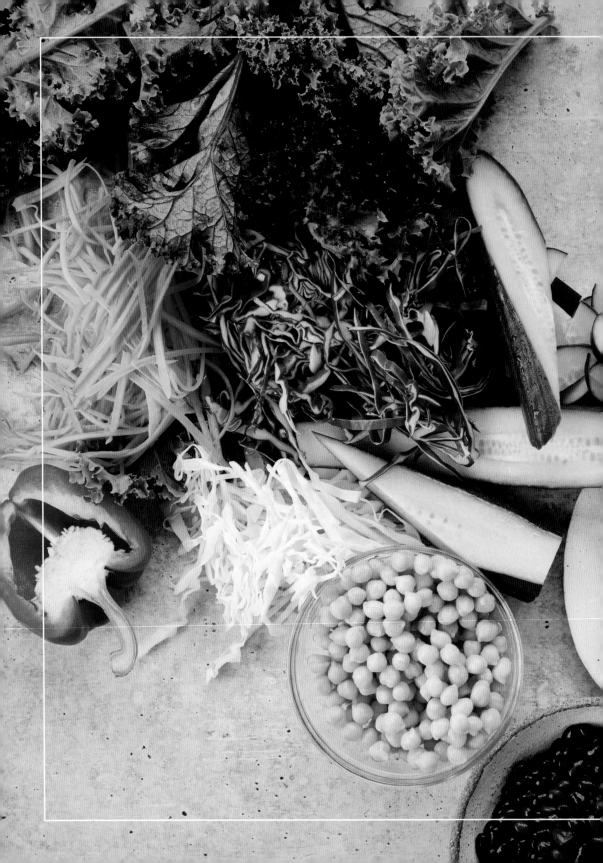

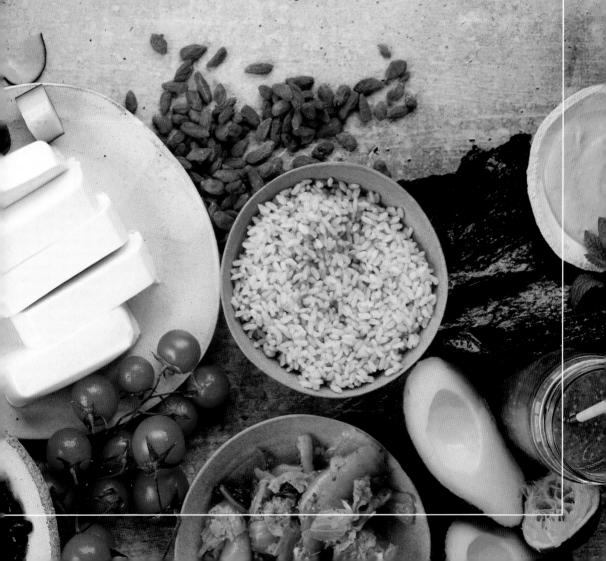

earth bowls and salads

*My Earth Bowls include a little of this, a little of that,
some sweet, some spice, some chew, and some crunch.
My favorite Earth Bowls are loaded with veggies and
topped with finger-licking sauce—satisfying, healthy, and
delicious! You can follow my Earth Bowl recipes, or use
them as a guide to DIY.*

YOUR DIY EARTH BOWL GUIDE

Here is a general guide for building your Earth Bowls, but really, there is no wrong way, so long as your ingredients are all Plant Over Processed!

1. **PICK YOUR LEAFY GREEN BASE.** Your base should be approximately 2 cups of one of the following, or a combination: romaine lettuce, spring greens, kale, arugula, baby spinach, Swiss chard, butter lettuce, mustard greens, or microgreens.

2. **CHOOSE YOUR VEGGIES FOR CRUNCH.** I recommend choosing two or three different raw veggies to add, about ¼ cup to ½ cup each. My favorite raw veggies for crunch are thinly sliced or roughly chopped carrots, bell peppers, cauliflower, radishes, red onions, beets, cucumber, and shredded pickled cabbage or pickled veggies.

3. **PICK YOUR PROTEIN.** Choose one or two proteins, ½ cup to 1 cup each. My favorite protein options include nuts, edamame, chickpeas, beans, tofu, and tempeh.

4. **PICK YOUR COMPLEX CARB.** Choose one or two, ½ cup to 1 cup of each. My favorites include roasted potato or sweet potato, cooked rice, roasted or steamed butternut squash, cooked peas, sautéed plantains, or cooked quinoa.

5. **PICK YOUR NOURISHING ADD-INS AS DESIRED.** Choose one to three, ¼ cup total. My favorites include sauerkraut, kimchi, diced avocado, daikon, seaweed, ginger, pumpkin seeds, hemp hearts, fresh herbs, and dulse flakes.

6. **SPRINKLE IN SOME SWEET.** This is optional, but you may also want to add a tablespoon of raisins, goji berries, dried blueberries, dried apple, or dried mango for a bit of chew and sweetness.

7. **PICK YOUR DRIZZLE.** See pages 186–189 for my favorite super simple dressings you can whip up in minutes and drizzle over your bowls.

Earth Bowls are incredibly adaptable, and any of the recipes below can be modified to create yummy burritos or pita sandwiches by simply taking a large tortilla shell or pita and filling with the listed ingredients.

MAKE A SALAD TOPPER JAR

Before we dive into the Earth Bowl and salad recipes in this next section, I want to share a simple hack that will take your salad game to the next level: Make a salad topper jar! This is a great way to give a flavorful kick to your salads and avocado toast, while also adding a nutritional boost.

1. Gather 1 cup baked pumpkin seeds (some of the healthiest seeds in the world, packed with nutrients, healthy fats, and antioxidants) and ½ cup hemp hearts (a great source of iron, potassium, and magnesium).

2. Use a blender or a knife and a cutting board to chop your pumpkin seeds and hemp hearts into a powder, or leave with some texture if you prefer.

3. Add ½ teaspoon salt and ½ teaspoon pepper and sprinkle everything into a mason jar for storage.

Your mixture is now ready to sprinkle onto salads, Earth Bowls, avocado toast, and even rice!

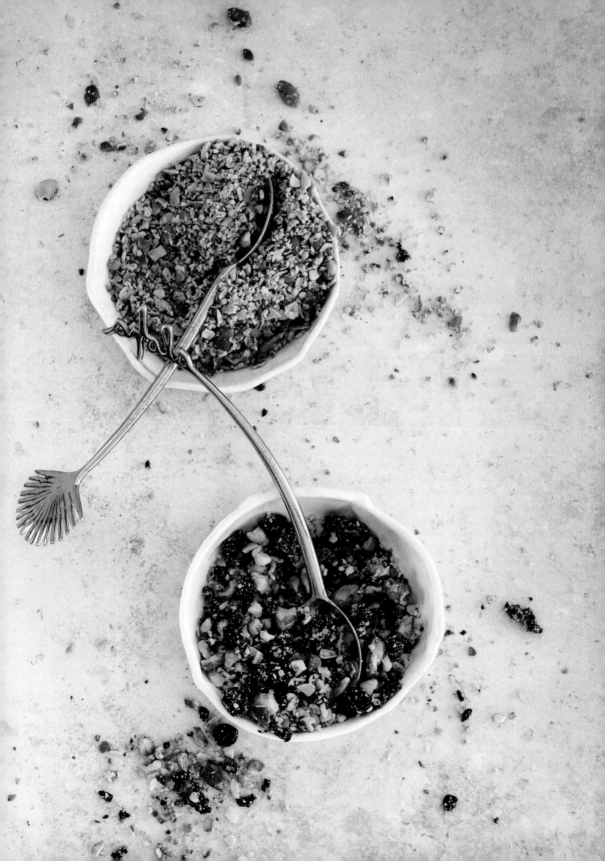

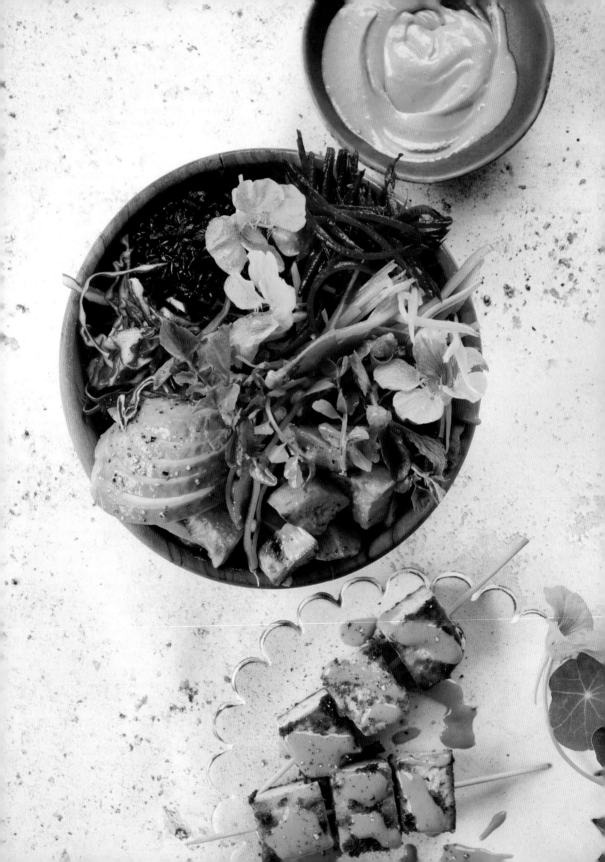

bali earth bowl

PREP TIME: 35 MINUTES • TOTAL TIME: 55 MINUTES • SERVES 2

Bali is one of my favorite island destinations to visit. It's a place full of life and culture, dramatic skies, and beautiful waves for days. You can't help but feel more alive just being there. Wherever you are in the world, treat yourself to a taste of Bali with the peanut sauce, black rice, and caramelized tofu in this bowl, inspired by traditional Balinese cuisine. The vegetables listed here are suggestions—feel free to pick and choose to make this bowl your own.

7 ounces tofu (firm or extra-firm)
1 large sweet potato
1 tablespoon extra virgin olive oil
Sea salt
1 cup North Shore Fusion Peanut Sauce (page 185)
¾ cup cooked black rice
½ cup finely shredded pickled purple cabbage (optional)
1 cup finely shredded carrots or julienned on a mandoline (optional)
1 cup finely shredded beets or julienned on a mandoline (optional)
1 cup sliced snap peas (optional)
1 avocado, sliced (optional)
¼ cup microgreens (optional)
½ cup baby leafy greens, such as sweet pea leaves, baby kale, or baby bok choy

1. Preheat the oven to 425°F. Line a baking sheet with parchment paper.

2. Blot the tofu dry with paper towels and cut into 2-inch cubes. Arrange on half of the prepared baking sheet.

3. Cut the sweet potato into 1-inch cubes and arrange on the other half of the same baking sheet.

4. Drizzle the sweet potato with the olive oil and sprinkle with salt. Drizzle half of the peanut sauce over the tofu and toss to coat well.

5. Bake the tofu and sweet potato for 25 to 30 minutes, turning each piece halfway through, until the tofu is caramelized and the sweet potato is soft in the middle.

6. Assemble each bowl with the black rice, tofu, sweet potato, and your choice of pickled cabbage, carrots, beets, snap peas, avocado, and microgreens. Finish with the baby leafy greens.

7. Drizzle with the remaining peanut sauce.

PREDOMINANTLY LIVING PLANT-BASED RECIPE

shawarma bowl

PREP TIME: 45 MINUTES • TOTAL TIME: 1 HOUR 15 MINUTES • SERVES 2

Channel the flavors of the Middle East with this delicious and healthy bowl. The roasted shawarma spiced cauliflower and chickpeas, fresh cucumbers, tomatoes, olives, fresh herbs, and red onions, all over a bed of leafy greens, are tied together with my Shawarma Drizzle!

2 teaspoons cracked black pepper, plus more for the salad
1 tablespoon curry powder
½ teaspoon red pepper flakes
¼ teaspoon garlic powder
Sea salt
1 (15-ounce) can chickpeas
2 tablespoons plus 2 teaspoons extra virgin olive oil
½ head cauliflower, cut into bite-sized florets
1½ tablespoons lemon juice, plus more to taste
1 cup cherry tomatoes, quartered
2 cucumbers, cut into ½-inch pieces
½ small red onion, thinly sliced, or ½ cup Pickled Red Onions (page 174)
¼ cup fresh cilantro or basil leaves, roughly chopped
¼ cup fresh mint leaves, roughly chopped
1 handful leafy greens (I like baby kale, but you can use any favorite)
½ cup Shawarma Drizzle (page 187)

1. Preheat the oven to 400°F.

2. In a small bowl, combine the black pepper, curry powder, red pepper flakes, and garlic powder and season with salt. This is your shawarma spice blend.

3. Drain and rinse the chickpeas and pat dry with paper towels. This will ensure the best texture from roasting. Toss the chickpeas with 1 tablespoon of the olive oil and spread evenly onto a baking sheet. Make sure there is space between the chickpeas for best texture results.

4. Toss the cauliflower with 1 tablespoon olive oil and about three quarters of the shawarma spice blend. Spread the cauliflower evenly onto a second baking sheet.

5. Place the baking sheets into the oven and roast until the chickpeas are golden brown and crisp and the cauliflower is soft when pierced with the end of a knife, about 30 minutes. Halfway through, toss the chickpeas and cauliflower to ensure even roasting.

NOTE: You can make double the amount of shawarma spice blend and store it in an airtight container. It's great thrown on any roasted veggies!

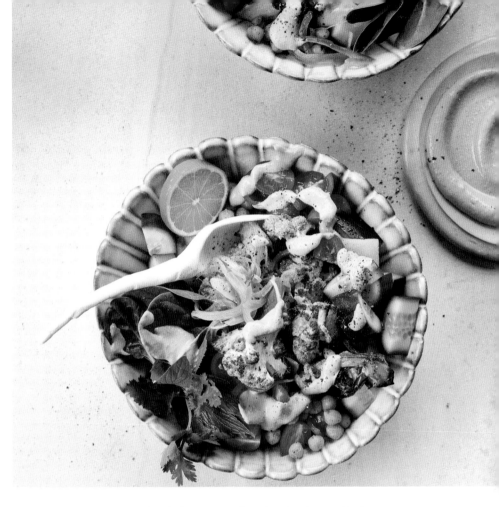

6. Spoon the chickpeas into a large bowl and toss with the remaining shawarma spice mix. (You can also toss the cooked cauliflower and chickpeas with some extra olive oil or lemon juice if you like.)

7. While the chickpeas and cauliflower are baking, place the tomatoes, cucumbers, red onion, cilantro or basil, and mint in a small bowl. Season with salt and black pepper, add the 1½ tablespoons lemon juice and the 2 teaspoons olive oil, and toss well. Set aside.

8. To assemble the bowls, add the leafy greens, roasted cauliflower, and chickpeas. Top with the tomato-cucumber mixture, drizzle with the shawarma drizzle, and serve.

PREDOMINANTLY LIVING PLANT-BASED RECIPE

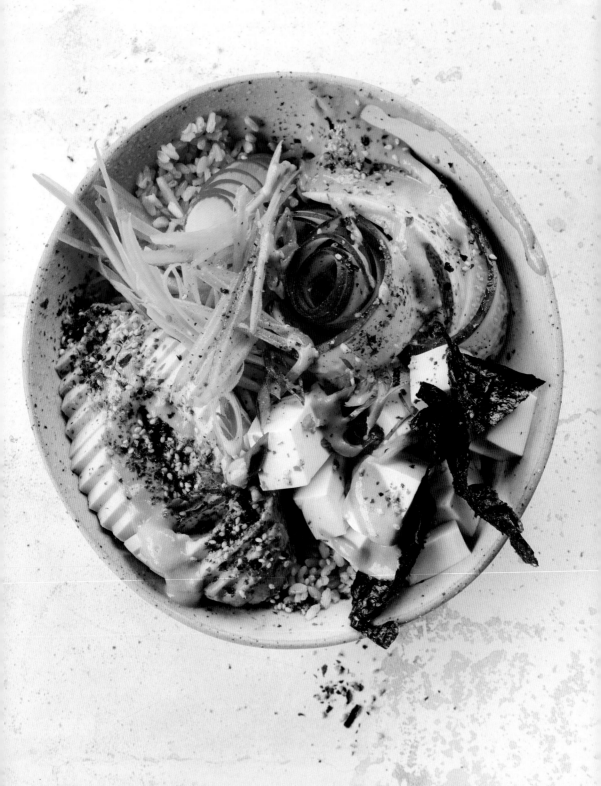

teri poke bowl

PREP TIME: 25 MINUTES • TOTAL TIME: 55 MINUTES • SERVES 2

Poke is a traditional native Hawaiian dish that dates back to when ancient Hawaiians feasted on freshly caught fish after massaging it with sea salt, seaweed, and crushed kukui nuts. Today's versions tend to be influenced by Asian cuisine, with ingredients that are marinated and served over a bed of warm rice. In this bowl, we're going to replace the fish with tofu and veggies—which is not traditional but is healthy and delicious—and flavor with teriyaki. You could also buy some nori seaweed and have fun wrapping these ingredients into hand rolls.

½ cup whole-grain rice
1¼ cups filtered water
2 teaspoons dry sake
1 (12-ounce) block firm tofu
½ cup Teriyaki Drizzle (page 186), plus extra for serving
1 tablespoon rice vinegar
1 tablespoon pickled ginger (optional)
¾ cup cooked edamame beans (optional)
¼ cup shredded carrot
¼ cup chopped or ribboned cucumber
1 ripe avocado, sliced
1 green onion, chopped
2 sheets nori seaweed, torn into pieces (optional)
1 tablespoon furikake seasoning (optional)

1. Pour the rice into a strainer and rinse until the water runs clear. Put the rice into a medium saucepan or rice cooker, pour in the water and sake, and give it a stir. If you are cooking the rice in a pan on the stovetop, cook over medium-high heat until the liquid has evaporated, about 15 minutes. Remove from the heat, cover, and let the rice sit for 15 minutes before checking that the rice is soft. Once the rice is done, fluff with a fork. If you are using a rice cooker, cook according to the machine's instructions, let the rice sit for 15 minutes, fluff it, and let cool before proceeding to the next steps.
2. While rice is cooking, cut the block of tofu into 2-inch cubes and coat with the teriyaki drizzle. (You can pan-fry or broil the tofu cubes for a crispy texture, if you like, or leave them uncooked.)
3. Transfer the cooked and cooled rice to a medium bowl. Add the vinegar and mix well.
4. To assemble the bowls, begin by adding an equal amount of rice to each bowl, then top with the remaining ingredients, sprinkling the nori and furikake over the rice or other ingredients, if using.
5. Top with the extra teriyaki drizzle and serve.

PREDOMINANTLY LIVING PLANT-BASED RECIPE

chipotle lime black bean bowl

add cheese ☺

PREP TIME: 20 MINUTES • TOTAL TIME: 1 HOUR 5 MINUTES • SERVES 2

This bowl is inspired by the flavors and nourishing ingredients of Mexico, including cilantro, lime, sweet potatoes, black beans, and avocado—and of course a dash of hot sauce. With flavors like these you're going to be salsa dancing around your house! When I prepare these bowls, I like to make an extra batch of black beans to use in other dishes throughout the week.

NOTE: You can roast the sweet potatoes and make the black bean mixture and pico de gallo ahead of time and store in the fridge so you have a simple meal you can throw together in no time.

1 sweet potato
2 tablespoons extra virgin olive oil
½ teaspoon paprika
Salt and freshly ground black pepper
1 (15-ounce) can black beans, drained and rinsed
¼ teaspoon chili powder
½ teaspoon garlic powder
Juice of 2 to 3 limes, plus 1 tablespoon lime juice
2 medium tomatoes, diced
½ cup diced white onion
½ cup finely chopped fresh cilantro leaves
½ cup corn kernels
1 cup shredded romaine lettuce
Toppings: cilantro leaves, diced avocado, tortilla strips, lime wedges
½ cup Chipotle Drizzle (page 189)

1. Preheat the oven to 425°F.
2. Cut the sweet potato into 1-inch cubes. Place in a medium bowl, toss with the olive oil and paprika, and season with salt and pepper. Roast for 40 minutes, or until lightly browned.
3. Put the black beans in a small saucepan. Place over medium heat and mix in the chili powder and garlic powder. Cook for 3 to 5 minutes, until the black beans are warm. Stir in the 1 tablespoon lime juice.
4. To make a quick pico de gallo, combine the tomatoes, onion, the juice of 2 limes, and the cilantro in a small bowl. Taste and add the juice of the third lime if needed. Set aside.
5. To build your bowls, divide the black beans, roasted sweet potatoes, corn, lettuce, and pico de gallo between bowls. Add any of the suggested toppings, drizzle with the chipotle drizzle, and serve.

PREDOMINANTLY LIVING PLANT-BASED RECIPE

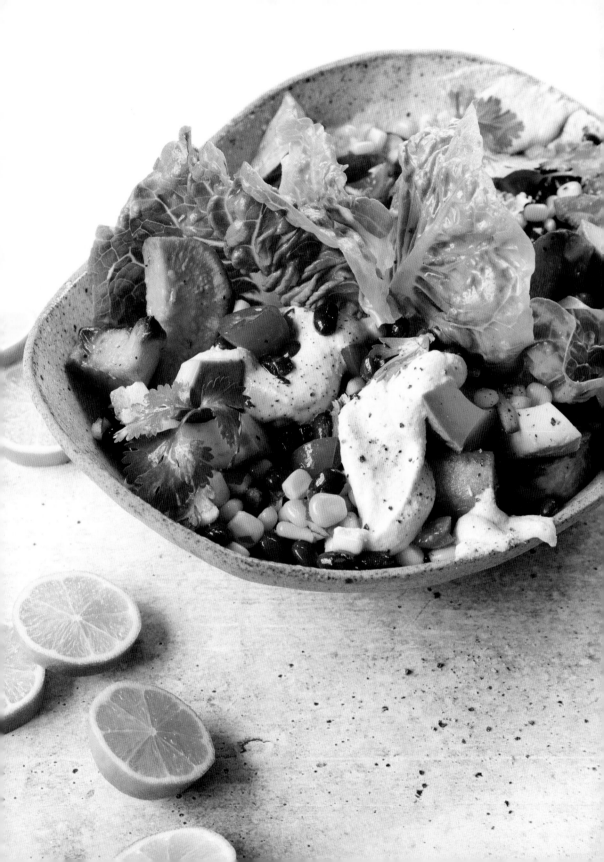

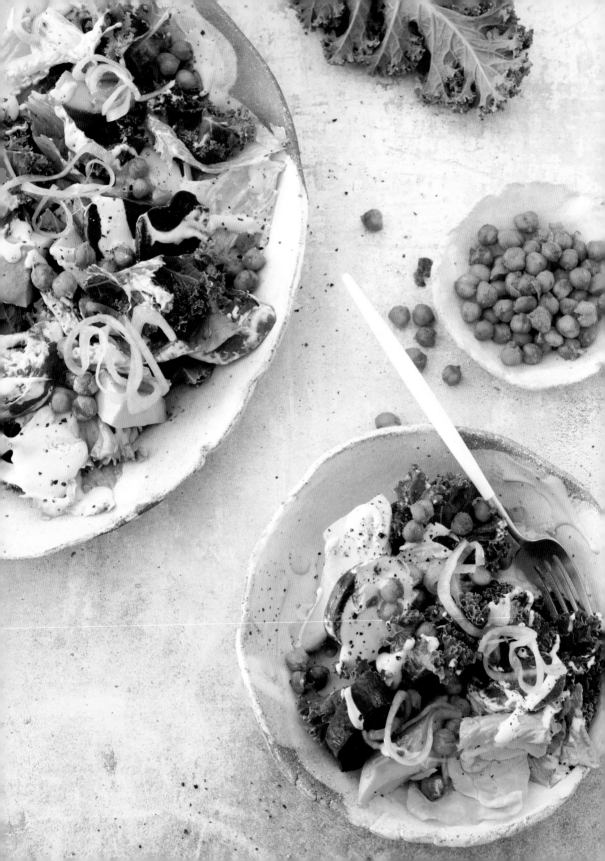

vegan caesar salad with chickpea croutons and roasted potatoes

PREP TIME: 10 MINUTES • TOTAL TIME: 40 MINUTES • SERVES 2

Traditional Caesar salad is one of the most popular salads of all time, but it can also be one of the least healthy. That's why I love this nutritious plant-based version, which still has tons of flavor. Chickpea croutons and macadamia Parmesan (see page 138) jazz it up, and tossing in some roasted potatoes makes it a hearty meal.

2 pounds red- or white-skinned potatoes
1 (15-ounce) can chickpeas
2 tablespoons extra virgin olive oil
1 teaspoon ground cumin
½ teaspoon ground turmeric
1 teaspoon garlic powder
Salt and freshly ground black pepper
1 to 2 cups curly kale
1 to 2 cups shredded romaine lettuce
Caesar Dressing (page 180)
Macadamia Parmesan cheese (see page 138)

1. Preheat the oven to 400°F.

2. Cut the potatoes into 1-inch chunks and place on a baking sheet.

3. Drain and rinse the chickpeas and pat dry with paper towels. Place on a second baking sheet.

4. Toss the potatoes in 1 tablespoon of the oil. Mix together ½ teaspoon of the cumin, ¼ teaspoon of the turmeric, and ½ teaspoon of the garlic powder and toss with the chickpeas. Season with salt and pepper. Toss the potatoes with the remaining 1 tablespoon oil, ½ teaspoon cumin, ¼ teaspoon turmeric, and ½ teaspoon garlic powder and season with salt and pepper.

5. Put both baking sheets in the oven and roast for 30 minutes. Remove from the oven and set aside.

6. Chop the kale and place it in a big bowl. Toss in the lettuce. Throw the roasted potatoes over the greens.

7. Just before serving, top with the Caesar dressing and toss. Sprinkle with the roasted chickpeas and macadamia Parmesan cheese.

PREDOMINANTLY LIVING PLANT-BASED RECIPE

vegan niçoise salad

PREP TIME: 10 MINUTES • TOTAL TIME: 45 MINUTES • SERVES 2

The first time I traveled to France the classic Niçoise salad quickly became one of my favorites. Now that I don't eat fish, I've created this vegan version that doesn't skip a beat on flavor and satisfaction! If you have never used chickpeas as a substitute for tuna, you are going to be amazed at what a great swap this is.

1 pound small red- or yellow-skinned potatoes
2 teaspoons extra virgin olive oil
Salt and freshly ground black pepper
1 (15-ounce) can chickpeas
6 cups baby kale or 1 head romaine lettuce, chopped
1 cup steamed green beans
¼ cup pitted green or kalamata olives
½ cup cherry tomatoes, halved
¼ cup Everyday OG Salad Dressing (page 180)

1. Preheat the oven to 400°F.

2. Cut the potatoes into halves or quarters and place on a baking sheet. Toss with the olive oil and season with salt and pepper.

3. Drain and rinse the chickpeas and pat dry with paper towels.

4. Spread the dried chickpeas over a separate baking sheet. Place in the oven with the potatoes and bake until the potatoes are fully cooked and the chickpeas are crisp, about 30 minutes. Remove from the oven. Place the chickpeas in a medium bowl and smash with a fork.

5. Place the kale in a salad bowl. Add the steamed green beans, olives, and cherry tomatoes and drizzle with the dressing.

6. Top with the chickpea tuna and baby potatoes and enjoy.

TIP: *You can use this method for making chickpea tuna to create a vegan tuna sandwich.*

PREDOMINANTLY LIVING PLANT-BASED RECIPE

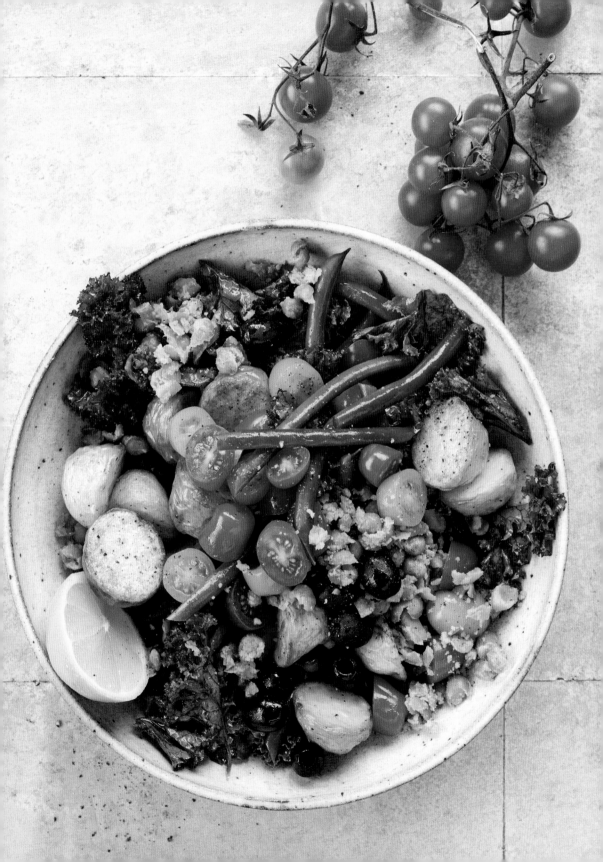

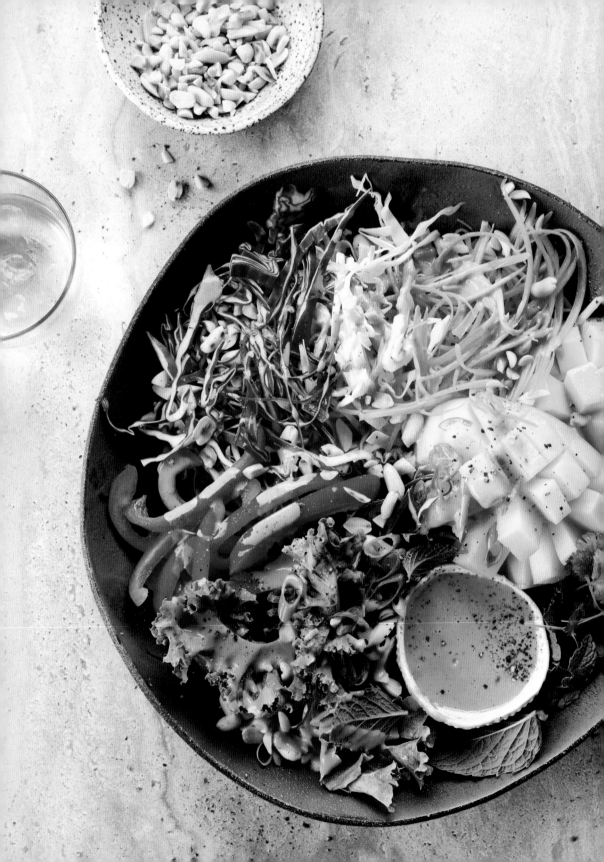

rainbow thai crunch salad

PREP TIME: 15 MINUTES • TOTAL TIME: 15 MINUTES • SERVES 2

This colorful salad is fun to look at and to eat. The peanut sauce, fresh mint, and roasted peanuts give it a Thai flair, and you can feel free to add rice noodles for an extra twist!

2 cups kale
12 ounces napa cabbage
8 ounces red cabbage
1 small red bell pepper
1 small carrot
¼ cup fresh cilantro leaves
10 fresh mint leaves
½ cup North Shore Fusion Peanut Sauce (page 185)
¼ cup crushed roasted peanuts
3 green onions, thinly sliced
1 ripe mango, diced (or substitute 2 tablespoons chopped dried mango)

1. Thinly slice the kale, cabbages, and bell pepper. Grate the carrot into shreds. Roughly chop the cilantro and mint and combine the chopped vegetables with half of the herbs.

2. Once you are ready to serve, toss the salad in the peanut sauce. Top with the crushed roasted peanuts, sliced green onions, mango, and the remaining herbs and enjoy.

LIVING PLANT-BASED RECIPE

rainbow rice paper rolls

PREP TIME: 15 MINUTES • TOTAL TIME: 30 MINUTES • SERVES 4

Oh, how I love this summery recipe, in any season. It's a variation of the Rainbow Thai Crunch Salad on page 121.

1 medium cucumber
2 medium carrots
¼ head small red cabbage
4 green onions
1 mango
1 avocado, sliced
8 rice paper wrappers
8 large leaves butter lettuce
½ cup fresh mint or Thai basil leaves
2 tablespoons crushed peanuts for topping
North Shore Fusion Peanut Sauce (page 185)

1. Slice the cucumber, carrots, cabbage, green onions, and mango into thin strips about 3 inches long. Set aside.

2. Fill a bowl wide enough to fit the rice paper wrappers with warm water. Soak 1 rice paper in the water for 15 to 30 seconds, until pliable. Put the rice paper on a counter or cutting board.

3. Arrange a few of the vegetables, leafy greens, and herbs in the center of the wrapper horizontally, starting with the whole lettuce leaves and ending with the avocado and mango.

4. Wrap like a burrito, folding the ends into the middle, then folding over from the center, tucking and rolling delicately but firmly. (If your first one falls apart, don't worry—it will still taste good, so no losses!) Repeat with the remaining wrappers and filling.

5. Cut the rolls in half so you can enjoy how beautiful they look and place on a serving platter. Sprinkle with crushed peanuts and drizzle with or dip in the peanut sauce.

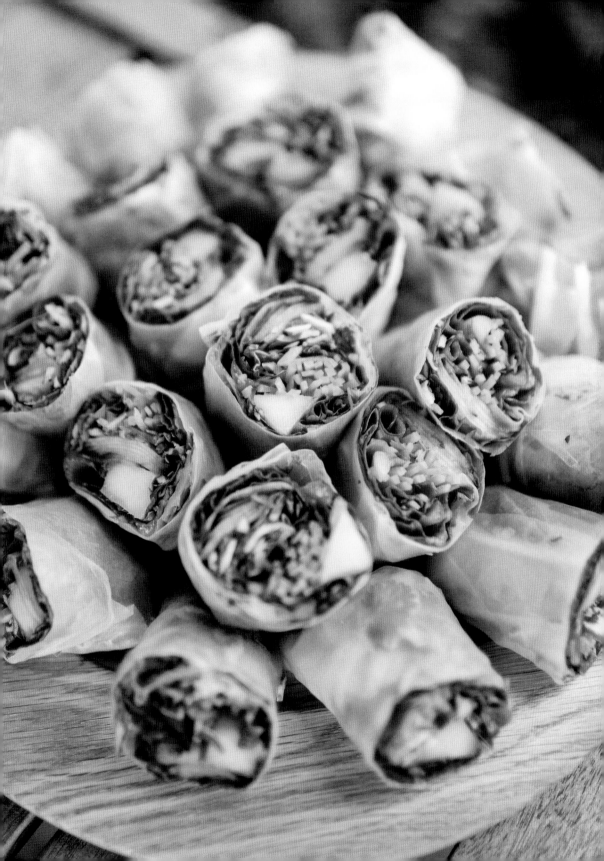

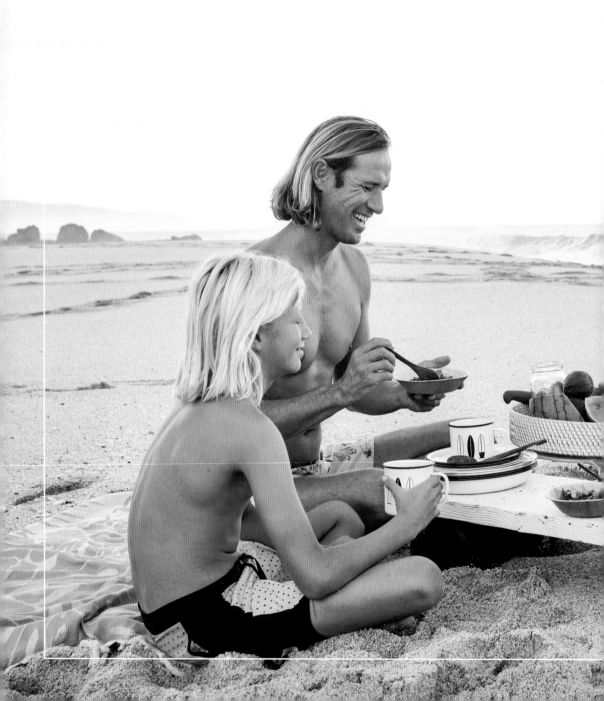

plant-based lunches and dinners

The healthy, delicious recipes in this section are meant to inspire you in the kitchen and to show you how easy it can be to make simple, satisfying meals for you and your family using plants! We are going to explore lots of flavor combinations to keep your taste buds entertained and your stomach feeling full and satisfied.

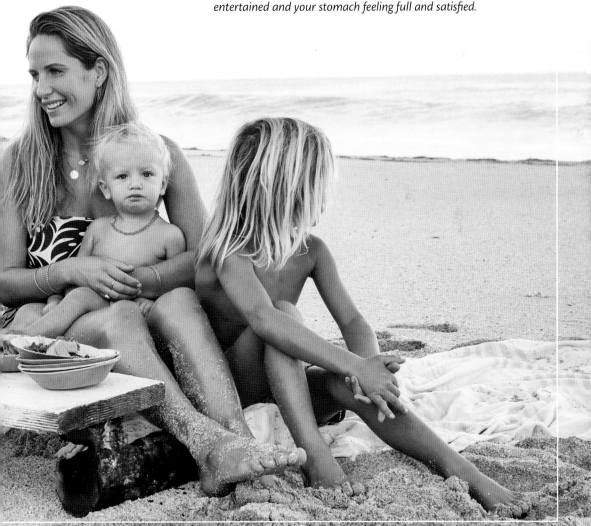

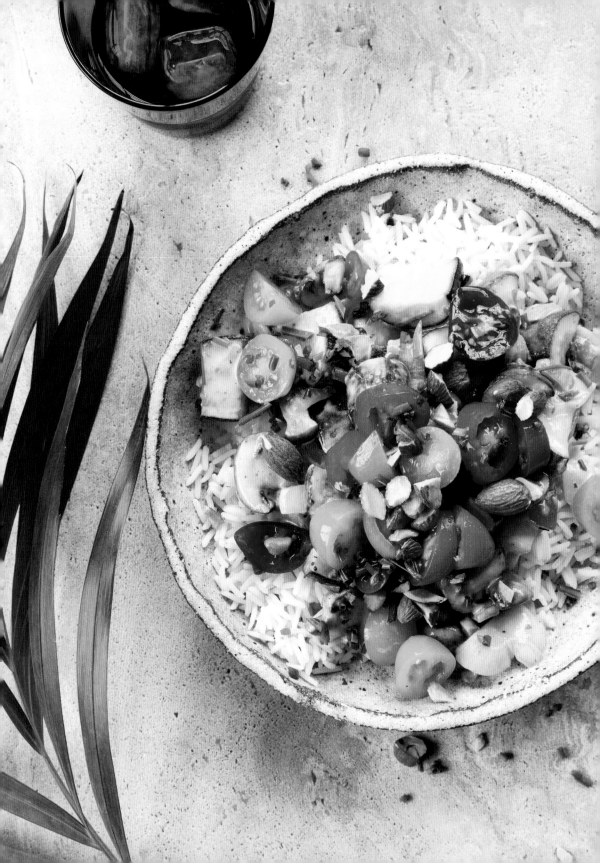

hawaiian haystacks

PREP TIME: 15 MINUTES • TOTAL TIME: 25 MINUTES • SERVES 4

This is a dish that my mom used to make for us back in Canada. In the dead of winter in Saskatchewan, we would pretend to be Hawaiian with this recipe (though it is not actually a Hawaiian dish!). Traditionally, it's made with chicken and a cream sauce poured over rice, with toppings like pineapple, cashews, wontons, and shredded coconut. My vegan version uses a cream sauce that's made with plant milk instead of cow's milk, vegetable stock instead of chicken stock, and peas, zucchini, and mushrooms instead of chicken—all served over a bowl of warm rice with the same toppings. (You can pick and choose from the list of suggested toppings.) It's a great way to feed a crowd!

1½ teaspoons extra virgin olive oil
½ white or yellow onion, chopped
1 cup chopped zucchini
1 cup halved button mushrooms
3 tablespoons vegan butter
1 tablespoon all-purpose gluten-free flour
2 cups unsweetened plant milk (I like oat milk)
1 tablespoon vegetable bouillon paste (or 1 stock cube dissolved in 2 tablespoons hot filtered water)
Salt and freshly ground black pepper
2 cups fresh or frozen peas
Steamed whole-grain rice or gluten-free toast for serving

TOPPINGS TO CHOOSE FROM:

Diced pineapple	Chopped almonds
Cashews	Chopped fresh chives
Wonton strips	Raisins
Shredded coconut	Diced avocado
Diced tomato	Currants

1. Heat the olive oil in a large saucepan over medium heat. Add the onion, zucchini, and mushrooms and cook until softened, about 5 minutes. Remove from the heat and set aside.

2. In a small saucepan, melt the vegan butter over low heat. Stir in the flour and cook for about 3 minutes, stirring while it bubbles, until it starts to thicken. Add the plant milk and vegetable bouillon paste and season with salt and pepper. Raise the heat to medium and stir for 1 to 2 minutes until everything comes to a low boil. Add the peas and cook for an additional 1 minute.

3. Serve over rice or with toast on the side. Pick and choose from the suggested toppings above—you can add all or none as you like!

COOKED PLANT-BASED RECIPE

sweet potato caesar burritos

PREP TIME: 10 MINUTES • TOTAL TIME: 45 MINUTES • SERVES 2

I love burritos because you can get creative with them with all kinds of flavor combinations. And you can pack them up easily and take them on the go! We make burritos for school lunches and to bring to the beach, and they get the kids to eat all sorts of healthy ingredients—like beans, rice, avocado, tomatoes, cabbage, mushrooms, and potatoes—without protest! And just so you know, every single Earth Bowl and salad can be rolled up and enjoyed as a burrito! Sometimes I want all the health wealth of a salad but can't be bothered to sit down and eat it with a fork, which is when the hefty burrito comes in handy. Just roll it up and all you need is one hand. Sweet!

2 medium sweet potatoes
1 (15-ounce) can chickpeas
2 tablespoons extra virgin olive oil
1 teaspoon ground cumin
½ teaspoon ground turmeric
1 teaspoon garlic powder
Sea salt and freshly ground black pepper
½ cup curly kale
½ cup roughly chopped romaine lettuce
Caesar Dressing (page 180)
2 tortillas

1. Preheat the oven to 400°F.
2. Cut the sweet potatoes into 1-inch chunks and place them on a baking sheet.
3. Drain and rinse the chickpeas and pat dry with paper towels. Place on a separate baking sheet.
4. Toss the sweet potatoes in 1 tablespoon of the oil. Mix together ½ teaspoon of the cumin, ¼ teaspoon of the turmeric, and ½ teaspoon of the garlic powder and toss with the sweet potatoes. Season with salt and pepper. Toss the chickpeas with the remaining 1 tablespoon oil, ½ teaspoon cumin, ¼ teaspoon turmeric, and ½ teaspoon garlic powder and season with salt and pepper.
5. Put both baking sheets in the oven and roast for 35 minutes, or until both the sweet potatoes and the chickpeas are golden brown. Remove from the oven and set aside.
6. Chop the kale, place in a serving bowl, and toss with the lettuce.
7. Add the chickpeas and sweet potatoes to the greens, toss with the Caesar dressing. To assemble the burritos, first warm the tortillas. Put half the filling in the middle of each tortilla. Fold in the ends of the tortillas over the filling and then fold in the tops and bottoms to completely close in the fillings.

PREDOMINANTLY LIVING PLANT-BASED RECIPE

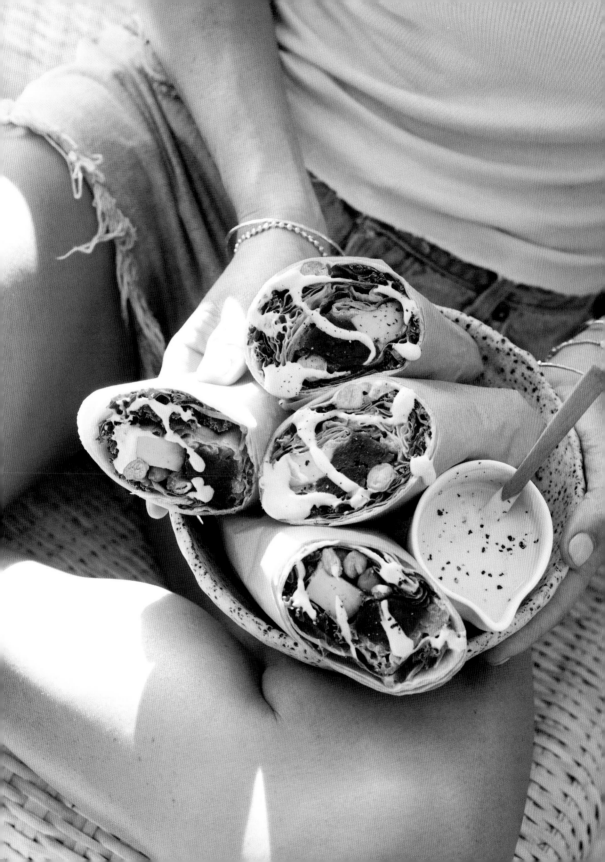

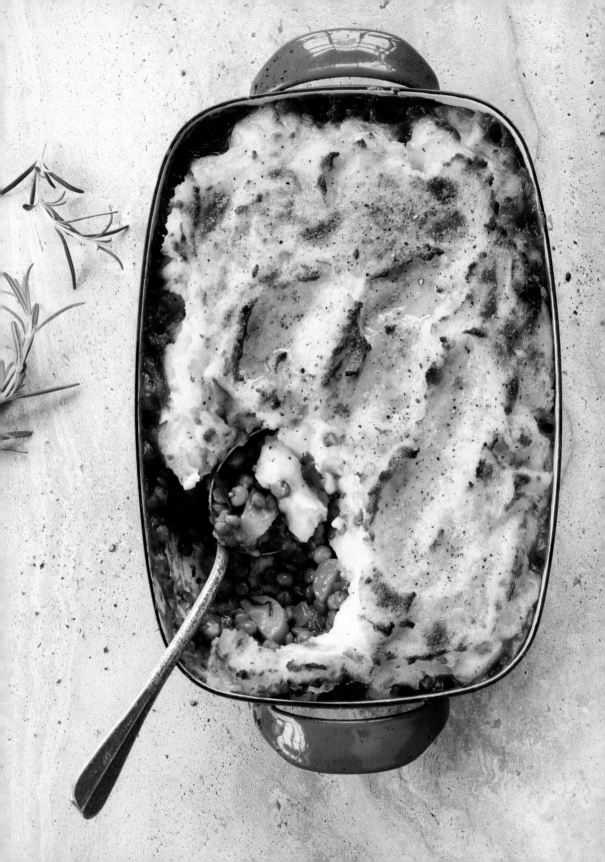

soul-hugging lentil shepherd's pie

PREP TIME: 45 MINUTES • TOTAL TIME: 1 HOUR 45 MINUTES • SERVES 6

This hearty plant-based casserole dish is a crowd-pleaser in my house. This is comfort food of the healthy variety, with protein-packed lentils and plenty of fiber and flavor. Oh, and who doesn't love a one-dish recipe for quick cleanup?

3 medium russet potatoes
2 tablespoons vegan butter or extra virgin olive oil
½ cup unsweetened plant milk
Sea salt and freshly ground black pepper
2 tablespoons extra virgin olive oil
1 cup chopped onion
4 medium carrots, finely diced
2 large cloves garlic, minced
3 cups cooked brown or green lentils
1 teaspoon ground turmeric
1 teaspoon ground cumin
2 tablespoons all-purpose gluten-free flour
2 teaspoons tomato paste
1 cup vegetable stock
1 teaspoon vegan Worcestershire sauce
2 teaspoons fresh rosemary leaves, chopped (or 1 teaspoon dried)
1 teaspoon fresh thyme leaves, chopped (or 1 teaspoon dried)
1 cup fresh or frozen peas

1. Preheat the oven to 400°F.

2. Peel the potatoes and cut into ½-inch chunks. Place in a medium saucepan and cover with cold water. Set over high heat, cover with a lid, and bring to a boil.

3. Remove the lid, lower the heat to maintain a simmer, and cook for 10 to 15 minutes, until you can easily smash a potato with a fork. Drain well.

4. In the same saucepan, melt the vegan butter over medium-low heat and mix in the plant milk. Return the potatoes to the saucepan and mash with a fork or potato masher until smooth. Season with salt and pepper and set aside.

5. While the potatoes simmer, prepare the filling. Heat a large sauté pan over medium-high heat and add the olive oil. Once

the oil is hot, add the onion and carrots and cook until the onion begins to soften, 3 to 4 minutes. Add the garlic and cook, stirring, for an additional 1 minute.

6. Add the cooked lentils, 1 teaspoon salt, ½ teaspoon pepper, the turmeric, and cumin and stir well. Add the flour, tomato paste, vegetable stock, Worcestershire sauce, rosemary, and thyme and stir to combine. Bring to a boil, reduce the heat to low, cover, and simmer for 10 to 12 minutes, until the sauce has thickened. Remove from the heat, add the peas, and stir to combine.

7. Spread the filling evenly into an 11 × 7-inch baking dish. Top with the mashed potatoes, spreading them evenly to the edges of the dish and forking across the top so you have some rough edges that will crisp up in the oven.

8. Bake for 25 to 35 minutes, until the potatoes just begin to brown. To crisp the top, turn the oven to broil and broil for an additional 3 to 5 minutes. Remove from the oven and allow to cool for at least 15 minutes before serving.

COOKED PLANT-BASED RECIPE

shem burger

PREP TIME: 45 MINUTES • TOTAL TIME: 1 HOUR 40 MINUTES • SERVES 6

As I've mentioned, Shem used to manage his family's chain of burger restaurants. One day, I challenged him to create an epic vegan burger recipe, and he accepted with open arms. After some trial and error, and getting the neighbors and kids to taste test, the Shem Burger was born. This burger was created in the spirit of love, community, and the belief that a vegan burger should not taste like birdseed! We love the gluten-free burger buns you can find in health food stores. Brioche buns are nice too, if you're not concerned about the gluten.

2½ tablespoons ground flaxseed
⅓ cup filtered water
2 tablespoons olive oil, plus extra for cooking the patties
3 cloves garlic, chopped
2 small white onions, chopped
2 tablespoons tomato paste
7 cups cooked brown lentils
½ cup cooked black beans
2 tablespoons finely grated beet
½ cup chopped button mushrooms
⅓ cup chopped green onions
2 tablespoons vegan Worcestershire sauce
¾ cup old-fashioned gluten-free rolled oats
¼ cup all-purpose gluten-free flour
Sea salt and freshly ground black pepper
6 gluten-free burger buns
Toppings: romaine or butter lettuce leaves, tomato slices, grilled onions, avocado, sprouts, vegan mayo, hummus

1. Combine the flaxseed and water in a blender or food processor and blend on high speed for 30 seconds to 1 minute, until smooth. Transfer to a bowl and set aside to use as the bonding agent for your burger patties.

2. Heat a large skillet over medium heat and add the olive oil. Once the oil is hot, add the garlic and onions and cook until softened and golden brown, 2 minutes. Add the tomato paste and mix well, reduce the heat to low, and cook for 5 minutes, or until the onions are cooked through.

3. Remove the skillet from the heat and stir in the lentils. Transfer to a large bowl.

4. Add half of the black beans and the grated beet to the bowl. Fold in the ingredients and mix well with a wooden spoon for 2 to 3 minutes to combine.

5. Transfer half of this mixture into a blender or food processor. Pulse for 15 to 30 seconds, until mostly smooth but with bits of onion, beans, and lentils visible. Remove from the blender or food processor and return to the bowl.

6. Add the mushrooms, green onions, Worcestershire sauce, and the remaining black beans. Mix the ingredients well with a spatula or with your hands for 2 to 3 minutes to combine. Add the flaxseed mixture and continue mixing until the ingredients are fully combined.

7. Add the oats and flour to the bowl and mix for another 2 to 3 minutes to combine. By now your ingredients should have a sticky and coarse consistency.

8. Cover and allow the mixture to chill in the fridge for 25 minutes to 1 hour. You want it to be cold so that it is easy to form patties without it sticking to your hands or your cooking surface.

9. For best results, form patties that are ¼ inch thick and 4 to 5 inches round (about the size of the palm of your hand). Once you have formed your patties, season them with salt and pepper on both sides.

10. Heat an oiled flat skillet or indoor or outdoor grill over medium-high heat. Add the patties and cook for 3 to 5 minutes on each side. They should be slightly crispy on the outside and soft in the inside.

11. Serve the burgers on the buns with your choice of toppings and condiments.

PREDOMINANTLY LIVING PLANT-BASED RECIPE

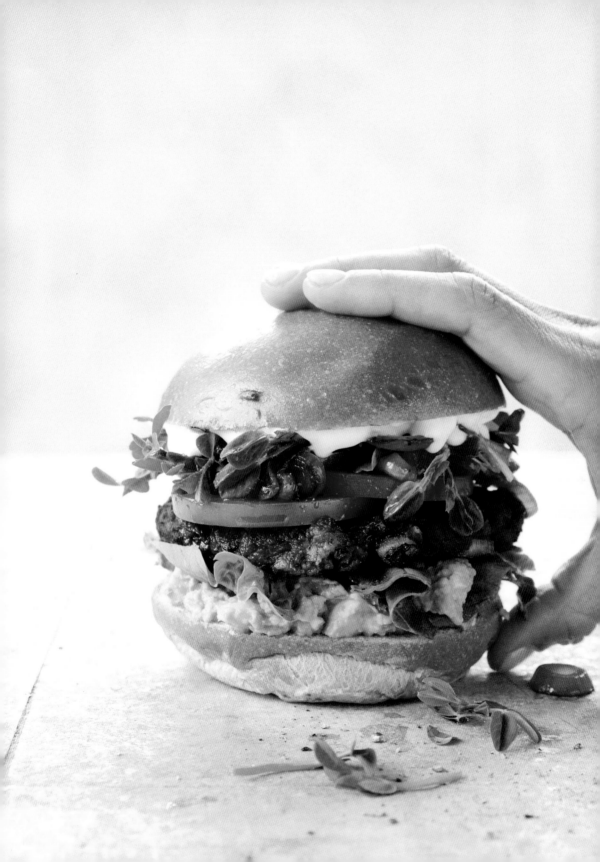

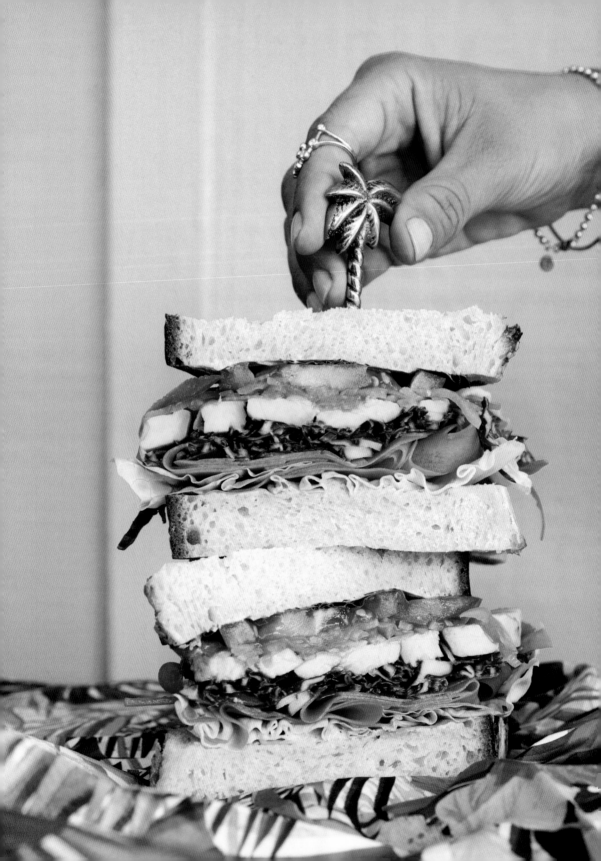

fully loaded sandwich

PREP TIME: 15 MINUTES • TOTAL TIME: 15 MINUTES • SERVES 1

Who says you need meat, cheese, and mayo to make a delicious, filling sandwich? Give this one a try and you will never turn your nose up at a fully veggie sandwich again! Not only is this sandwich stacked with yummy ingredients, it's also loaded with vitamins, minerals, fiber, and protein!

2 slices gluten-free bread of choice (I love sourdough)
4 leaves romaine lettuce
1 small carrot
¼ cucumber
½ ripe avocado
½ large tomato
1 teaspoon stone-ground or Dijon mustard
1 tablespoon Bomb Hummus (page 168; optional)
Sea salt and freshly ground black pepper
¼ cup sliced red cabbage
¼ cup broccoli sprouts, or any favorite sprout
1 tablespoon Pickled Red Onions (page 174)

1. Toast the bread and let cool before adding the toppings to prevent it from getting soggy.

2. Tear the lettuce into pieces the size of your bread. Julienne or shred the carrot. Thinly slice the cucumber. Cut thick slices of the avocado and tomato.

3. Spread the mustard and hummus, if using, on each slice of bread.

4. Build your sandwich: Top one slice of bread with half of the lettuce leaves, then the carrot, cucumber, salt and pepper, red cabbage, avocado, sprouts, tomato, pickled red onions, then the remaining lettuce, and top with the second slice of bread.

5. Wrap tightly in parchment paper and slice in half to see all the colorful layers of your healthy veggie sandwich!

PREDOMINANTLY LIVING PLANT-BASED RECIPE

spaghetti with simple garlic basil tomato sauce and macadamia parmesan

PREP TIME: 30 MINUTES • TOTAL TIME: 45 MINUTES • SERVES 4

Spaghetti is a no-brainer when it comes to filling hungry bellies with something satisfying, quick, and inexpensive! Making your own sauce will not only save you from the additives and sugar in many store-bought brands. It will also taste better and it only takes a few minutes to make. And the macadamia Parmesan looks and even tastes a bit like Parmesan!

1 (1-pound) package gluten-free spaghetti
1 teaspoon sea salt, plus more for seasoning
1 tablespoon extra virgin olive oil
1 small yellow onion, roughly chopped
1 tablespoon minced garlic
2 (14.5-ounce) cans crushed tomatoes (I like fire-roasted, but any kind will do)
1 teaspoon dried oregano
½ cup fresh basil leaves, chopped, plus whole leaves for serving
Freshly ground black pepper
¼ cup macadamia nuts

1. Bring a large pot of water to a boil. Add the pasta and the salt and cook according to the package instructions.

2. While the pasta cooks, heat the olive oil in a large skillet over medium heat. Add the onion and cook until softened, 1 to 2 minutes, then add the garlic and cook for another 3 minutes, until the onion is translucent and the garlic aroma has strengthened.

3. Add the crushed tomatoes and oregano to the skillet and cook for 15 minutes, or until slightly reduced. Remove from the heat and add the chopped basil. Season with extra salt and pepper. If you like your sauce to have a smooth texture, transfer the mixture to a food processor or blender and process for a minute or so, until smooth. For a chunky sauce, leave it as is.

4. Add the pasta to the sauce and divide among serving bowls.

5. Grate the macadamias over the pasta for your macadamia Parmesan.

COOKED PLANT-BASED RECIPE

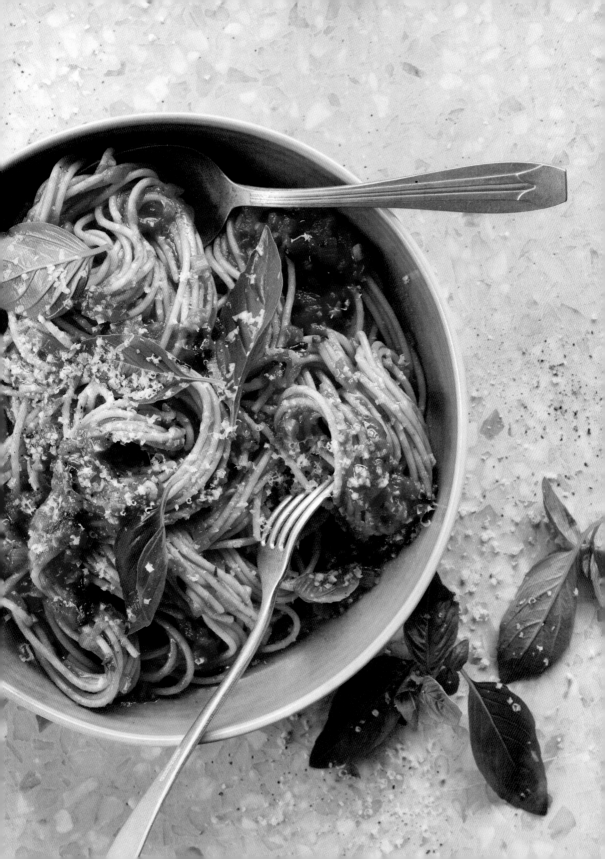

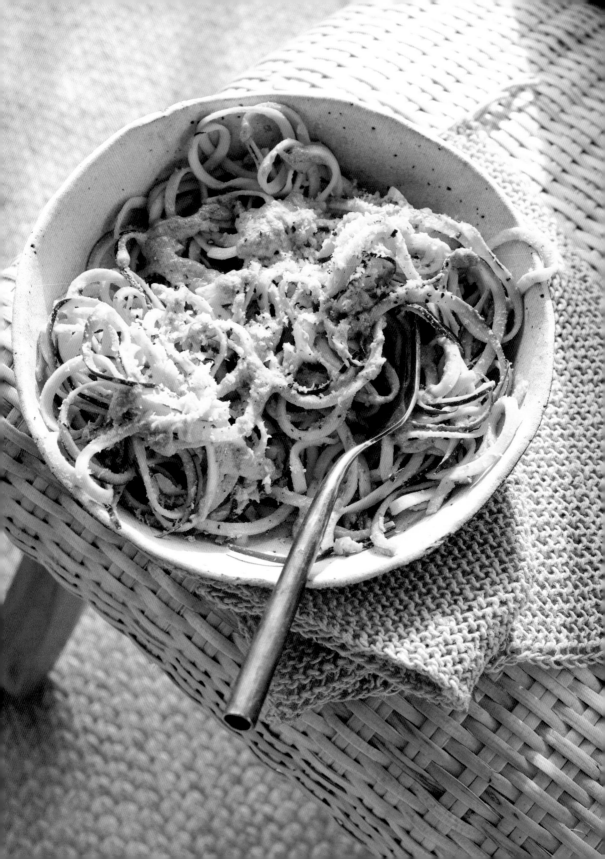

pesto zoodles

PREP TIME: 5 MINUTES • TOTAL TIME: 10 MINUTES • SERVES 2

Pesto zoodles are a fun way to fill up on vegetables. You will be packing in nutrients and flavor in a way that even the kids will love. Zoodles make for a great raw salad topper too!

2 medium zucchinis
1 tablespoon extra virgin olive oil
1 clove garlic, minced
Sea salt and freshly ground black pepper
¼ cup Macadamia Nut Pesto (page 178)

EQUIPMENT:
Vegetable spiralizer (If you don't have a spiralizer, you can use a vegetable peeler or just cut thin strips with a knife. It won't look the same, but it will still taste great!)

1. Slice the ends off one of the zucchinis and place the flat end on your spiralizer. Turn the spiralizer to create zucchini noodles. Repeat with the second zucchini.

2. Heat the olive oil in a large skillet over medium heat. Add the garlic and cook for 30 seconds.

3. Add the zucchini noodles and toss for 1 minute just to warm through but keep their texture, then turn off the heat. The zoodles will still be firm but slightly transparent and heated through.

4. Season with salt and pepper, toss in the macadamia nut pesto, and enjoy immediately.

COOKED PLANT-BASED RECIPE

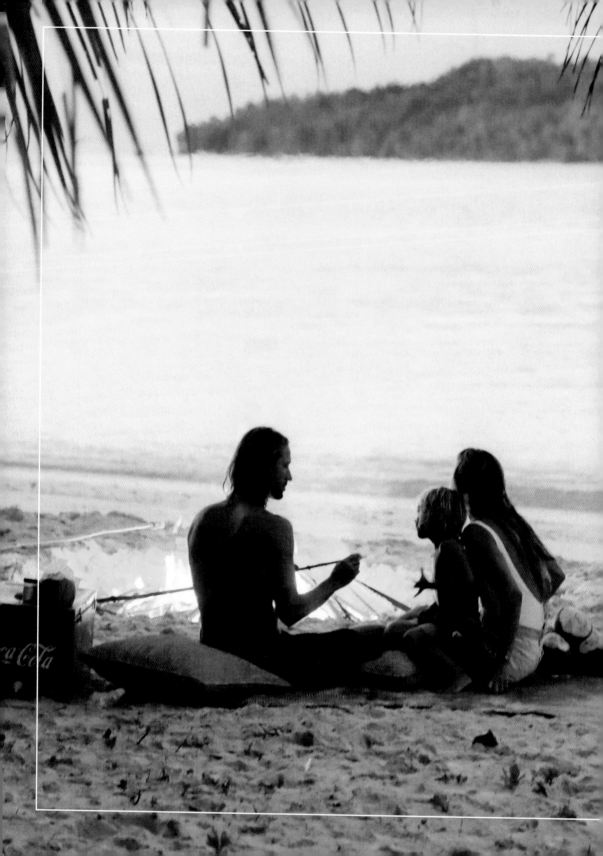

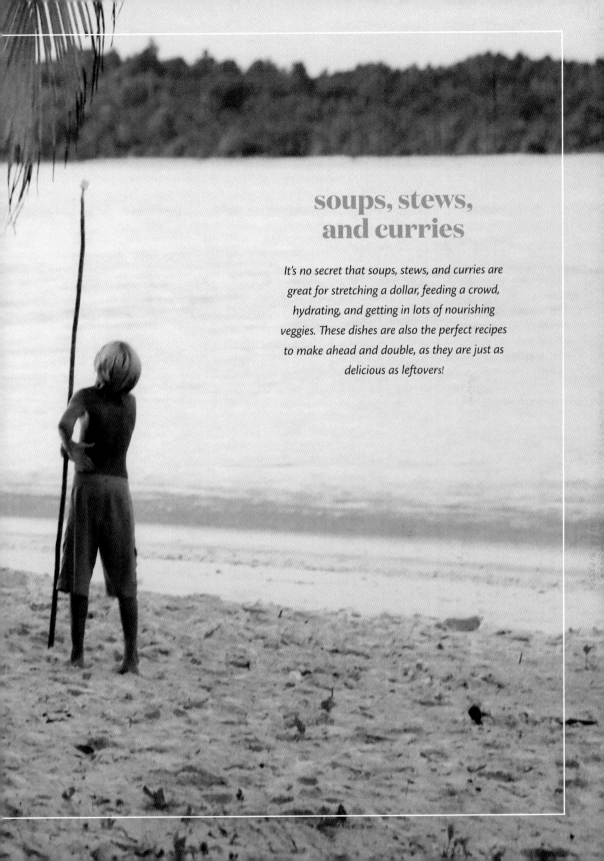

soups, stews, and curries

It's no secret that soups, stews, and curries are great for stretching a dollar, feeding a crowd, hydrating, and getting in lots of nourishing veggies. These dishes are also the perfect recipes to make ahead and double, as they are just as delicious as leftovers!

beach bum chili

PREP TIME: 25 MINUTES • TOTAL TIME: 1 HOUR 10 MINUTES • SERVES 6 TO 8

After a long day at the beach surfing and playing in the shore break, there's no better meal to come home to than a warm bowl of chili! When my husband and his six brothers were growing up, they'd spend all day surfing together, and when the sun went down this was their favorite meal to enjoy. This is a simple, delicious dish to warm your belly and soul, and I promise you, it has so much flavor, you won't even miss the meat.

2 tablespoons extra virgin olive oil
1 medium red onion, chopped
1 red bell pepper, chopped
2 medium carrots, chopped
2 celery stalks, chopped
½ teaspoon sea salt
1 tablespoon minced garlic (about 4 cloves)
1 tablespoon chili powder
2 teaspoons ground cumin
1½ teaspoons smoked paprika
1 teaspoon dried oregano
2 (15-ounce) cans diced tomatoes (I like fire-roasted, but any kind will do)
2 (15-ounce) cans black beans, drained and rinsed
1 (15-ounce) can kidney or pinto beans, drained and rinsed
2 cups vegetable broth or filtered water
1 bay leaf
½ cup chopped fresh cilantro leaves, plus more for garnish
1½ teaspoons red wine vinegar or lime juice, or to taste
Toppings and garnishes: chopped cilantro, sliced avocado, tortilla chips, Nach-Yo Everyday Cheese Sauce (page 177)

1. In a large heavy-bottomed pot, heat the olive oil over medium heat until shimmering. Add the onion, bell pepper, carrots, celery, and ¼ teaspoon of the salt. Stir to combine and cook for about 10 minutes, stirring occasionally, until the vegetables are tender and slightly browned.

2. Add the garlic, chili powder, cumin, smoked paprika, and oregano and cook, stirring constantly, for about 1 minute, until well combined and the garlic has a chance to cook.

3. Add the tomatoes and their juices, the black beans, kidney beans, vegetable broth, and bay leaf. Stir to combine and bring the mixture to a simmer. Continue cooking, stirring occasionally and reducing the heat as necessary to maintain a gentle simmer, for 30 minutes. Remove the chili from the heat.

4. Transfer 1½ cups of the chili to a blender, making sure to get some of the liquid. Securely fasten the lid and blend until smooth (watch out for hot steam), then pour the blended mixture back into the pot. Alternately, you can blend the chili briefly with an immersion blender or mash it with a potato masher until it reaches a thicker consistency. Add the chopped cilantro and vinegar or lime juice. Add the remaining ¼ teaspoon salt and combine well.

5. Divide the mixture among individual bowls and serve with your choice of toppings and garnishes. The chili will keep in the refrigerator for up to 4 days, or you can freeze it for up to 1 month.

COOKED PLANT-BASED RECIPE

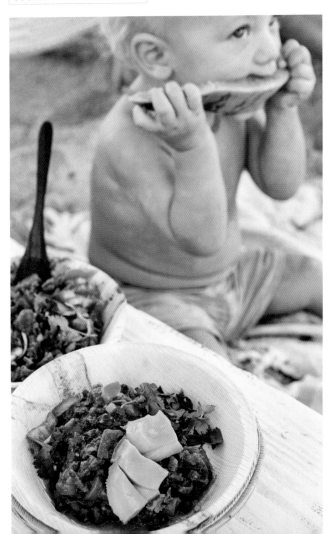

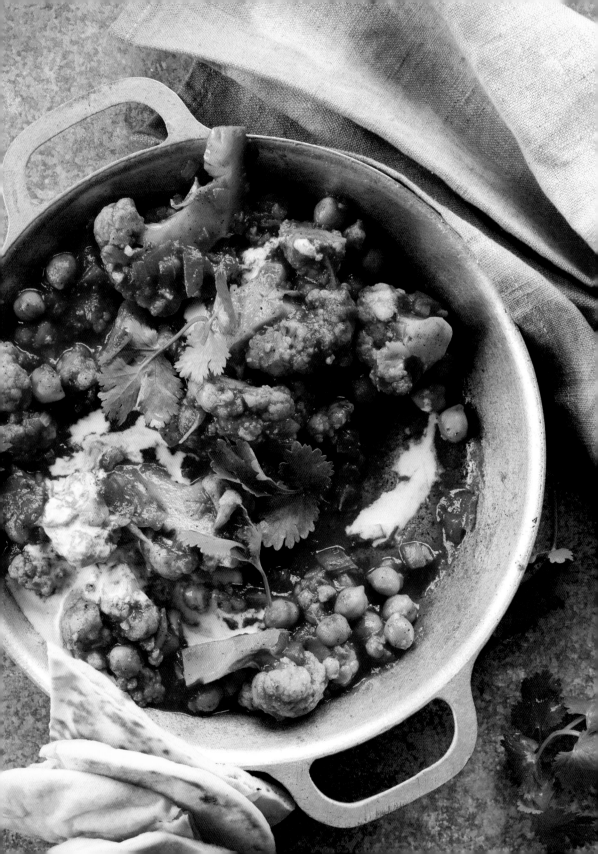

spice up your life cauliflower chickpea masala

PREP TIME: 10 MINUTES • TOTAL TIME: 30 MINUTES • SERVES 4

This rich, warming soup, inspired by the flavors of India, is full of veggies, herbs, and spices that are sure to make your mouth dance. If you like bold flavors, this one is for you!

½ teaspoon ground cumin
½ teaspoon ground turmeric
½ teaspoon smoked paprika
¼ teaspoon cayenne pepper (optional)
½ teaspoon sea salt, plus more as needed
Freshly cracked black pepper
1 tablespoon extra virgin olive oil or coconut oil
1 medium onion, chopped
3 cloves garlic, minced
1½ teaspoons grated fresh ginger or 1 teaspoon ground ginger
1 medium head cauliflower, cut into small florets
1 (15-ounce) can chickpeas, drained
1 (15-ounce) can no-sugar-added tomato sauce
1 cup vegetable broth or filtered water
½ cup canned unsweetened coconut milk
¼ cup fresh cilantro leaves, roughly chopped
Brown basmati rice and gluten-free naan flatbread for serving

1. In a small bowl, combine the cumin, turmeric, paprika, cayenne, salt, and black pepper to taste. This is your masala spice mix!

2. In a large, heavy saucepan, heat the olive or coconut oil over medium-high heat. When the oil is shimmering, add the onion, garlic, and ginger and cook over medium heat until the onion is softened, about 5 minutes. Stir in the spice mix and continue to cook for another minute.

3. Add the cauliflower to the pan and continue to cook until it begins to soften, about 10 minutes. Add a splash of water if needed if the spices are starting to burn.

4. Add the chickpeas, tomato sauce, and vegetable broth or water and stir to combine. Simmer over medium-low heat for 10 to 15 minutes, then turn off the heat and stir in the coconut milk. Add more salt if needed. Stir in the cilantro.

COOKED PLANT-BASED RECIPE

5. Serve with a bowl of basmati rice and some flatbread.

hug me lentil soup

PREP TIME: 10 MINUTES • TOTAL TIME: 1 HOUR 5 MINUTES • SERVES 6

A rich and hearty medley of vegetables, lentils, and herbs, this is the perfect comfort food, and it's a soup that I grew up on. Now here I am packing it in school lunches for my own kids! Lentils are one of the world's healthiest foods, packed with complex carbs, fiber, folate, and iron.

1 tablespoon extra virgin olive oil
1 medium white onion, chopped
4 cloves garlic, chopped or crushed
2 small carrots, chopped
3 celery stalks, chopped
2 russet potatoes, peeled and cut into 1-inch cubes
2 teaspoons ground cumin
2 bay leaves
2 (15-ounce) cans diced tomatoes
6 cups vegetable stock, plus more if needed
2 cups uncooked brown or green lentils
Sea salt and freshly ground black pepper
1 tablespoon lemon juice
Leaves from 1 bunch fresh parsley or cilantro, roughly chopped

1. In a large soup pot, heat the olive oil over medium-high heat. Add the onion, garlic, carrots, celery, potatoes, and cumin and cook until the vegetables are almost tender, about 10 minutes. Add a bit of water if needed to prevent sticking.

2. Add the bay leaves, tomatoes with their juices, vegetable stock, and lentils. Bring to a gentle boil, stirring occasionally, and boil until the lentils and potatoes are soft, then reduce the heat and simmer for 10 minutes. Add more stock if you'd like your soup to have a thinner consistency.

3. Transfer 1 to 2 cups of the soup to a blender and blend (or use an immersion blender), then add it back to the soup for added body. Season with salt and pepper.

4. Add the lemon juice and parsley or cilantro and serve.

COOKED PLANT-BASED RECIPE

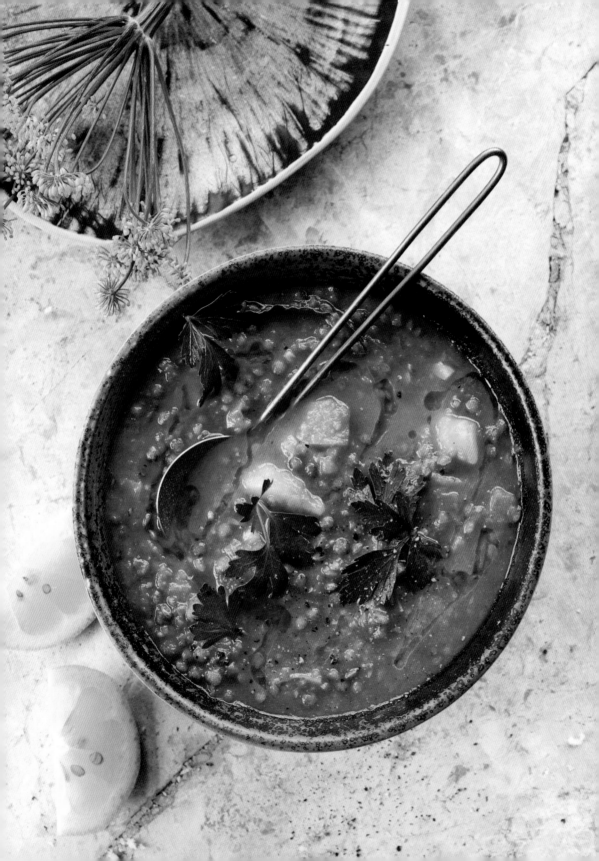

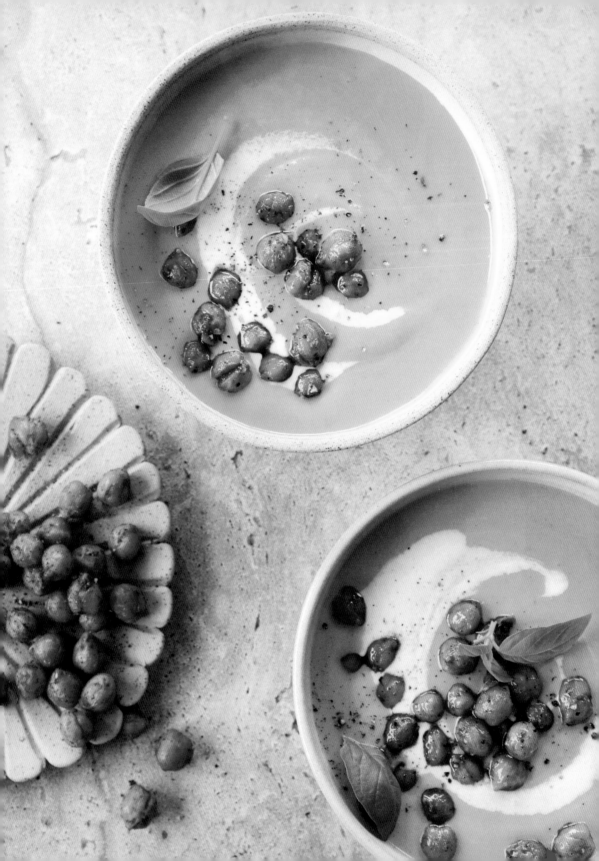

golden healing power soup

PREP TIME: 10 MINUTES • TOTAL TIME: 30 MINUTES • SERVES 6

A perfect blend of healing ingredients—turmeric, coconut milk, onion, and garlic—this soup will reduce inflammation, give you an antioxidant boost, and warm you from the inside out. It's perfect for nourishing your body and making you feel whole.

1 tablespoon extra virgin olive oil
½ white onion, chopped
2 cloves garlic, chopped
1 small head cauliflower, chopped into bite-sized florets
Pinch cayenne pepper (optional)
1 tablespoon ground turmeric
4 to 5 cups canned unsweetened coconut milk
1 teaspoon sea salt, plus more to taste
1 tablespoon lemon juice
Freshly ground black pepper
½ cup fresh basil leaves, finely chopped
Curried Chickpea Croutons (page 164)
Roasted cauliflower for garnishing (optional)
Coconut milk for garnishing (optional)

1. Heat the olive oil in a large soup pot over medium heat. When the oil is shimmering, add the onion, garlic, cauliflower, cayenne, if using, and turmeric. Cook for 10 minutes, or until fragrant.

2. Add half of the coconut milk and 1 teaspoon of the salt, bring to a simmer, and simmer until the cauliflower softens, about 10 minutes.

3. Transfer the soup to a blender and blend to a creamy consistency. (I blend in my Vitamix on high speed for 1 minute.)

4. Return to the soup pot over medium heat and gradually add more coconut milk until you reach your desired consistency. Simmer for 3 to 5 more minutes.

5. Add the lemon juice and additional salt and black pepper to taste and serve garnished with the basil, chickpea croutons, roasted cauliflower, and a swirl of coconut milk, if using.

COOKED PLANT-BASED RECIPE

red coconut curry

PREP TIME: 30 MINUTES • TOTAL TIME: 45 MINUTES • SERVES 6

Thai coconut curry is one of my absolute favorites. Whenever one of our family members has a cold someone in our extended family is bound to bring over some Thai soup, so the love runs deep. One year we decided to play around with learning Thai cuisine, and this is one of our favorites we keep coming back to. Bursting with flavor and packed with nutrients, you'll want to double this recipe every time!

1 tablespoon coconut oil
1 large yellow or white onion, finely chopped
1 cup fresh shiitake mushrooms, stemmed and halved
¼ cup Thai red curry paste
1 tablespoon vegan Thai chili paste
1 teaspoon ground turmeric
4 stalks lemongrass, minced or cut into 2-inch pieces (stem only; optional)
Thumb-sized piece of ginger, sliced into thin strips
2 cups vegetable stock or filtered water
2 (14-ounce) cans unsweetened coconut milk
4 kaffir lime leaves (optional)
4 medium carrots, chopped into small bite-sized pieces
4 potatoes (any variety you like), chopped into small bite-sized pieces
1 cup fresh or thawed frozen peas
¼ cup lemon or lime juice
1 cup fresh cilantro leaves, roughly chopped
Whole-grain rice for serving

1. Place a large pot over medium heat and add the coconut oil. When the oil is hot, add the onion and mushrooms with a splash of water. Add the curry paste, chili paste, turmeric, lemongrass, if using, and ginger and cook, stirring frequently, until the vegetables are softened, about 10 minutes. Add the vegetable stock or water and coconut milk and bring to a simmer.

2. Add the kaffir lime leaves, if using, the carrots, and potatoes. Return to a simmer, then reduce the heat to low and simmer covered until the potatoes and carrots are softened, about 10 minutes. Stir in the peas, lemon or lime juice, and cilantro and remove from the heat.

3. Serve over rice.

COOKED PLANT-BASED RECIPE

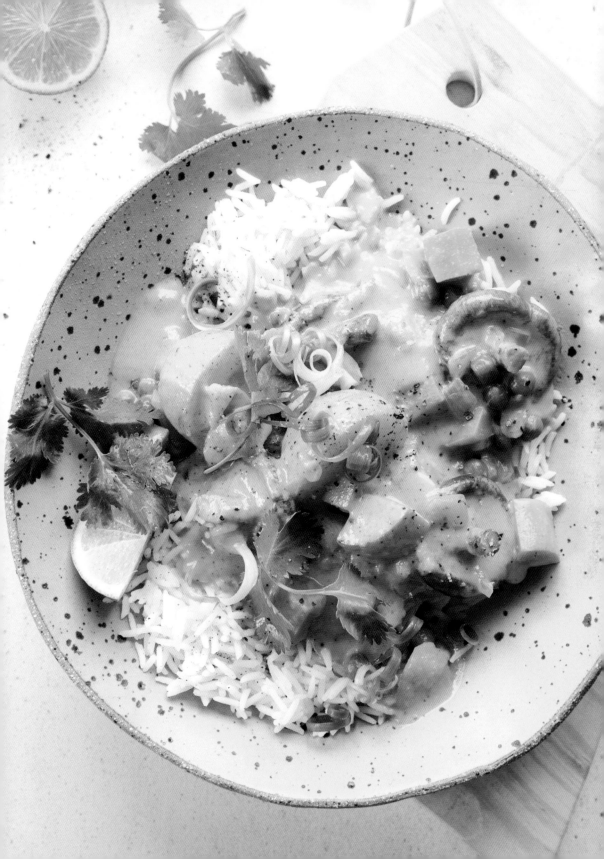

creamy no-cheddar broccoli soup

PREP TIME: 30 MINUTES • TOTAL TIME: 40 MINUTES • SERVES 4

I call this a magic soup because it tastes just like real rich cheddar-y cheese, but it is 100 percent plant-based. It's nourishing and delicious, especially on a cold, rainy day!

¼ cup extra virgin olive oil
1 large yellow onion, chopped
2 celery stalks, chopped
4 large carrots, chopped
4 cloves garlic, minced
1 large potato, peeled and chopped
3 to 4 cups vegetable broth
2 cups unsweetened oat milk (or 1 cup cashews blended with 1 cup filtered water until creamy)
2 cups cauliflower florets, cut into bite-sized pieces
2 cups broccoli florets, cut into bite-sized pieces
½ cup nutritional yeast
1 cup fresh or frozen peas
Sea salt and freshly ground black pepper
1 tablespoon lemon juice (optional, but adds another level of flavor)
½ cup fresh basil leaves
Gluten-free sourdough croutons (see Note)

1. Heat the olive oil in a large soup pot over medium-high heat. Once the oil is shimmering, add the onion and cook for 3 minutes, or until it starts to soften. Add the celery and carrots and cook for another 5 minutes, until the vegetables are soft. Add the garlic and cook, stirring, for an additional 1 minute.

2. Add the potato and vegetable broth, bring to a simmer, then reduce the heat and simmer for 10 minutes.

3. Add the oat milk, cauliflower, and broccoli. Simmer for 5 minutes, or until softened and the potatoes and carrots are soft enough to press a fork through.

4. Transfer 2 cups of the soup to a blender, making sure you get some of the liquid,. Add the nutritional yeast, and blend on high speed for 30 seconds, or until smooth.

NOTE: *There are two ways to make your sourdough croutons. The first way is to take a thick slice of your favorite gluten-free sourdough bread and toast it in the toaster. Once toasted extra-crunchy but not burnt, roughly chop it into big bite-sized pieces, drizzle with a little olive oil, season with a dash of garlic powder, salt, and pepper, and it's done. The second way is to roughly chop your sourdough bread slice, then toss the pieces with a little olive oil and toast in a skillet over medium-high heat for 1 to 2 minutes, tossing back and forth until golden.*

COOKED PLANT-BASED RECIPE

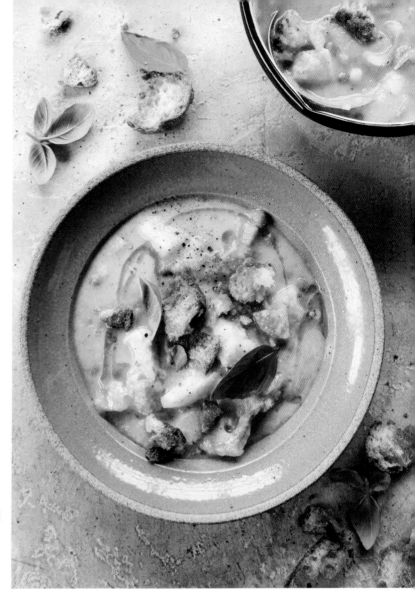

5. Pour the blended soup back into your soup pot. This is how you make it creamy! You can blend more and make it even thicker, but this is the ratio I like.

6. Add the peas, season with salt and pepper, and add the lemon juice, if using.

7. Portion the soup into soup bowls and top with the basil and homemade sourdough croutons.

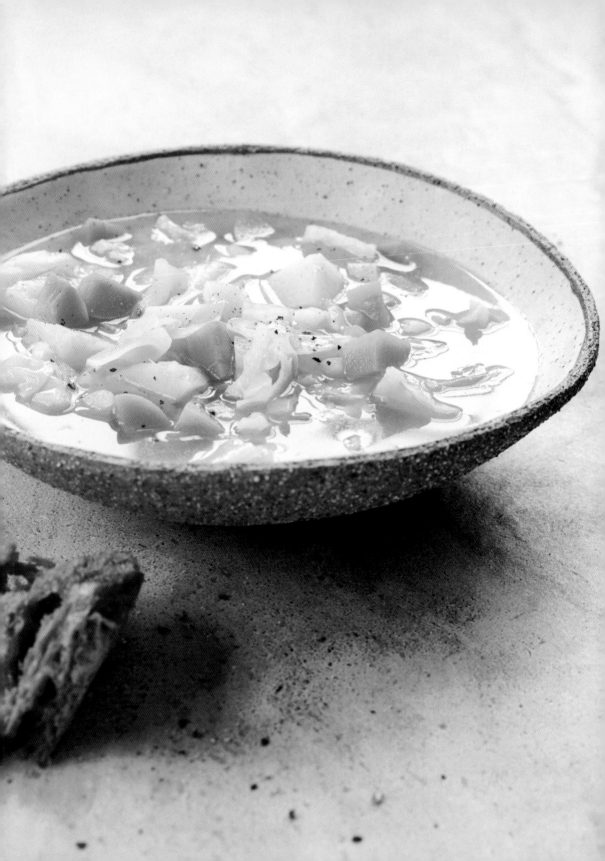

save your dollars soup

PREP TIME: 15 MINUTES • TOTAL TIME: 35 MINUTES • SERVES 6

This is a soup that I probably have made more than any other dish on this planet! It's a stretch-your-dollar, throw-a-few-ingredients-into-a-pot-and-be-done, and surf-a-little-longer kind of soup. All you need for this soup is cabbage, an onion, a couple carrots, and a potato or two! So simple yet so good!

1½ tablespoons extra virgin olive oil
1 large yellow onion, chopped
4 medium carrots, chopped into bite-sized pieces
1 to 2 large Yukon Gold potatoes chopped into bite-sized pieces
4 cups vegetable broth
1 small head green cabbage, roughly chopped
½ teaspoon freshly ground black pepper
Sea salt

1. Heat the olive oil in a soup pot over medium heat. Once the oil is shimmering, add the onion and cook for 5 minutes. Add the carrots and potatoes and cook for 2 to 3 more minutes, until the vegetables begin to soften.

2. Add the vegetable broth, raise the heat to medium-high, and add the cabbage. Make sure the cabbage is submerged under the liquid, bring to a simmer, then lower the heat and simmer for 10 to 15 minutes, until all the vegetables are softened.

3. Add the pepper, season with salt, and enjoy.

COOKED PLANT-BASED RECIPE

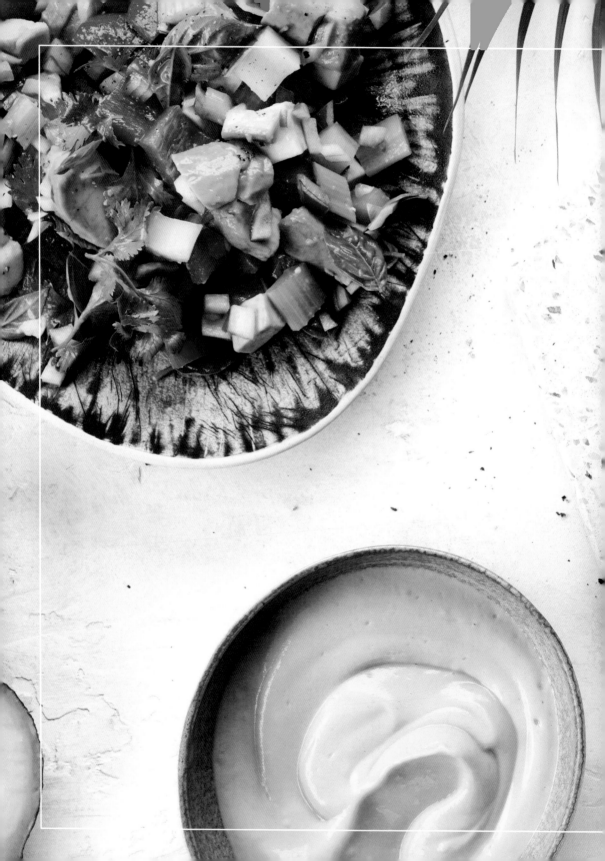

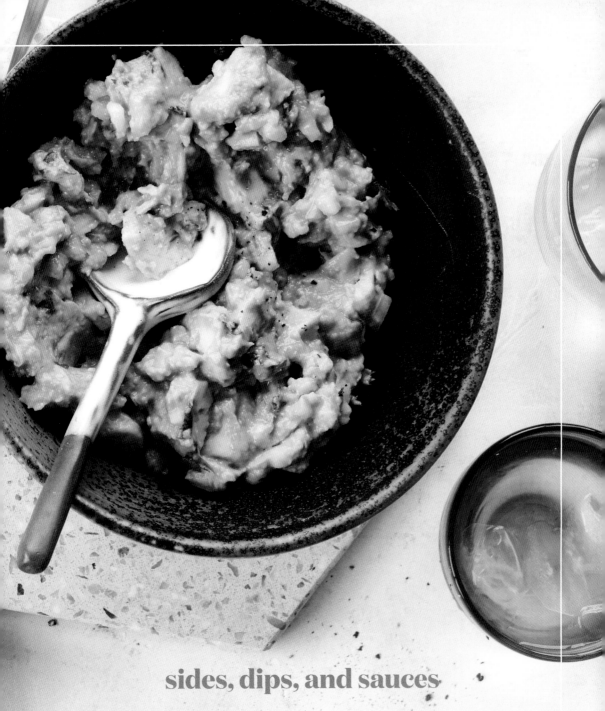

sides, dips, and sauces

A great dip or sauce can make an ordinary meal something special. Many store-bought sauces and dips are loaded with additives, extra sugars, and thickeners—things that we want to avoid—so let's make our own! And let's not forget about the sides in this section, which are so yummy that you may be tempted to make some as a main course!

lemon pepper potato fries

PREP TIME: 10 MINUTES • TOTAL TIME: 45 MINUTES • SERVES 2 TO 3

Potatoes have gotten a bad rap over the years. But the truth is that if they are not deep-fried or whipped together with loads of cheese and butter, potatoes are one of nature's most easily digestible foods, and they are full of nutrients. So let's ditch the notion that fries are bad for you, because these oven-baked fries are a whole lot of good.

3 large Yukon Gold potatoes
2 tablespoons extra virgin olive oil
Pinch Himalayan salt
1 teaspoon garlic powder
1 teaspoon lemon pepper seasoning (optional)
Grated lemon zest (optional)
Dips: organic ketchup, Vegan Sour Cream (page 184), or Avo Whip (page 170)

1. Preheat the oven to 400°F.
2. Slice the potatoes into fry shapes or wedges.
3. Cook the potatoes in a pot of boiling water until almost cooked through but still firm when poked with a fork, about 10 minutes. Drain and pat the potatoes dry.
4. Place the parcooked potatoes into a baking dish. Drizzle with the olive oil and sprinkle with the salt, garlic powder, and lemon pepper seasoning, if using. Roast in the oven for 20 minutes, or until the fries are crispy and golden, turning the fries over midway for even crisping.
5. Remove the fries from the oven and sprinkle with lemon zest for a bit of extra boogie.
6. Serve with your choice of dips and perhaps with a big salad alongside.

COOKED PLANT-BASED RECIPE

sweet potato cinnamon wedges

PREP TIME: 5 MINUTES • TOTAL TIME: 35 MINUTES • SERVES 2 TO 3

These highly nutritious delicious poppers are crunchy and slightly caramelized on the outside and soft and warm on the inside. They're the perfect addition to any Earth Bowl, or as a side to go with any dish. Sweet potatoes are known to promote gut health, enhance brain function, and support the immune system!

2 large sweet potatoes
2 teaspoons ground cinnamon
Sea salt and freshly ground black pepper
1 tablespoon coconut sugar

1. Preheat the oven to 425°F. Line a baking sheet with parchment paper.
2. Cut the sweet potatoes into equal-sized wedges and place on the lined baking sheet. Sprinkle the wedges with the cinnamon and salt and pepper to taste.
3. Place the baking sheet in the oven and bake for 30 minutes, or until the potatoes are tender and golden brown and crisp on the outside.
4. Pull out of the oven, sprinkle with the coconut sugar, and enjoy.

COOKED PLANT-BASED RECIPE

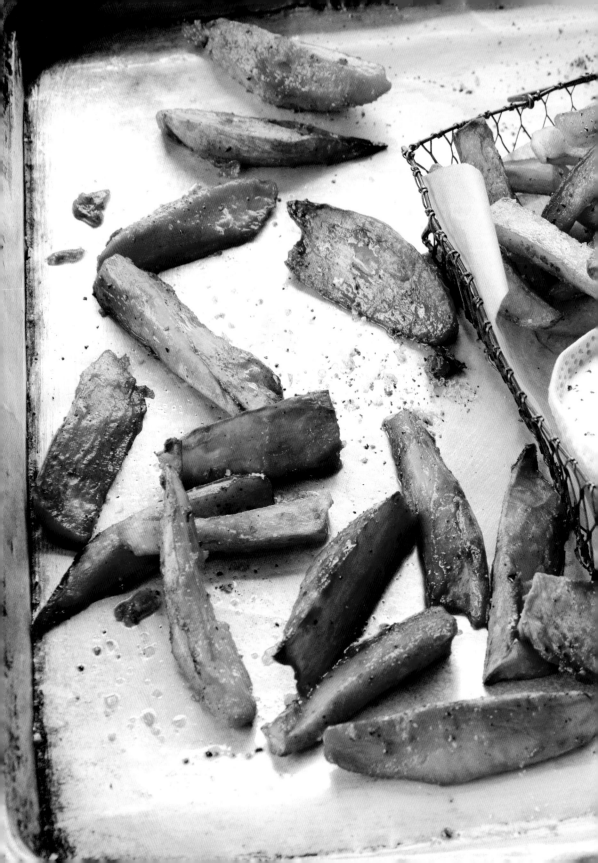

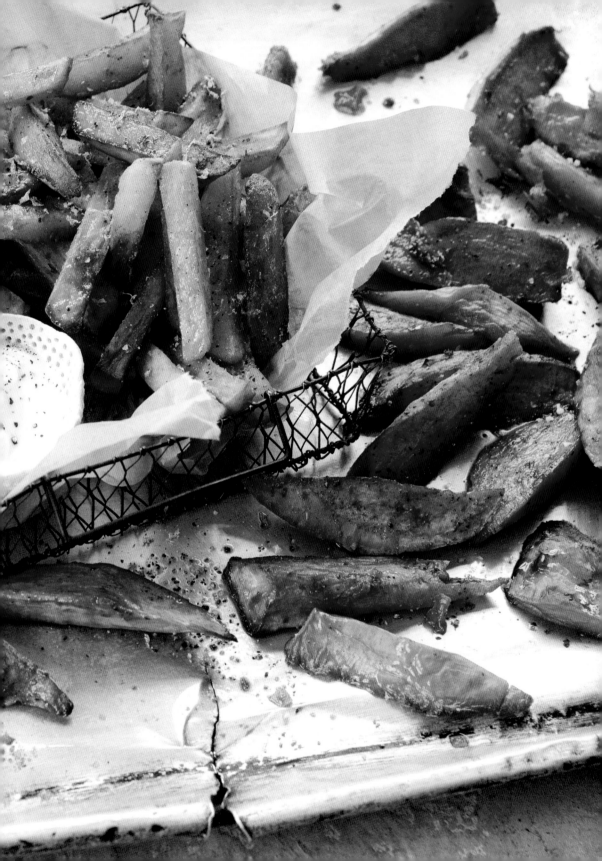

curried chickpea croutons

PREP TIME: 4 MINUTES • TOTAL TIME: 35 MINUTES • SERVES 2 TO 4

These are great as a protein-packed snack or side dish, and they add the perfect hearty crunch to any salad!

1 (15-ounce) can chickpeas
2 tablespoons red curry paste or 1 tablespoon curry powder
1 tablespoon extra virgin olive oil
1 tablespoon gluten-free tamari sauce
Pinch sea salt

1. Preheat the oven to 400°F. Line a baking sheet with parchment paper.

2. Drain and rinse the chickpeas and pat dry with paper towels.

3. In a medium bowl, combine the chickpeas, curry paste or curry powder, olive oil, tamari, and salt. Toss to coat.

4. Spread in an even layer on the prepared baking sheet and roast for 30 minutes, stirring every 10 minutes, until the chickpeas look toasted.

TIP: *To save time, you can cook the chickpeas in a nonstick skillet over medium heat, tossing frequently, for 10 minutes, or until toasted.*

COOKED PLANT-BASED RECIPE

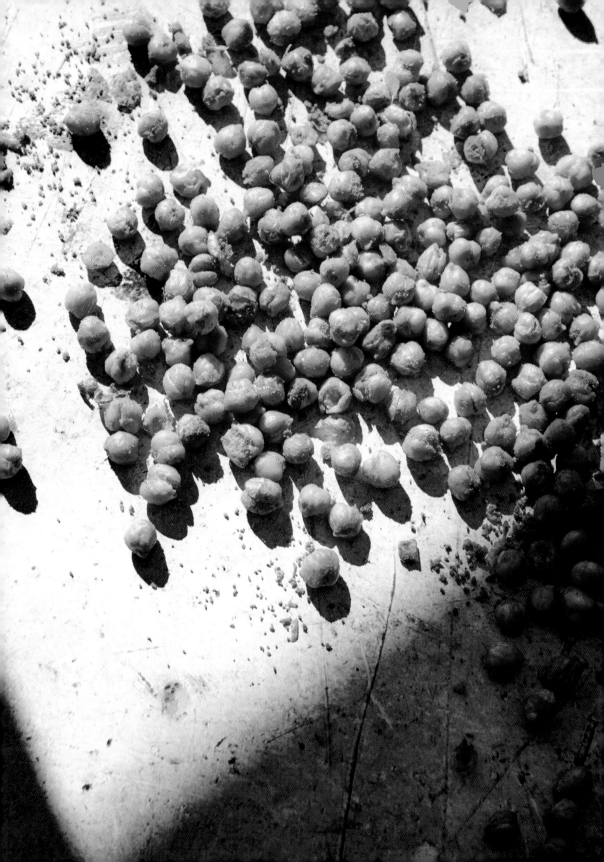

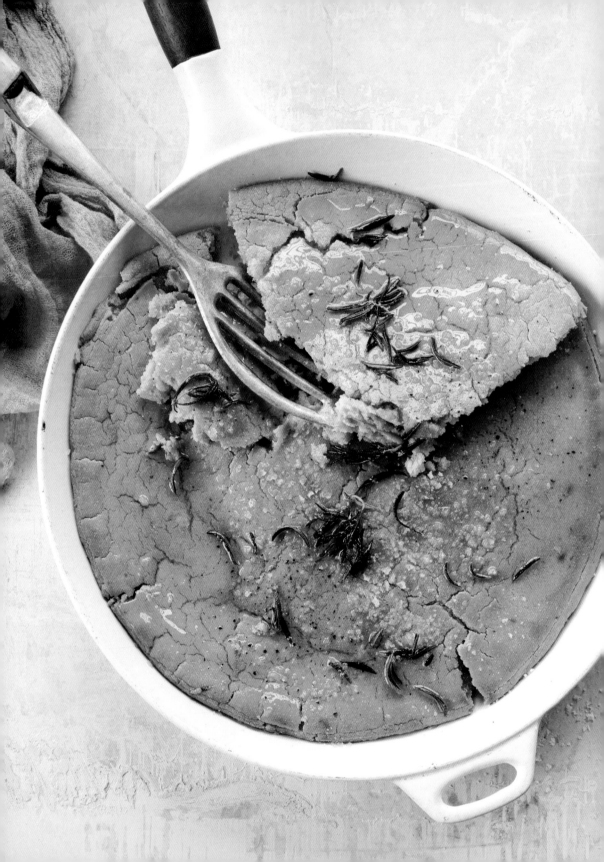

socca (gluten-free chickpea flatbread)

PREP TIME: 10 MINUTES • TOTAL TIME: 25 MINUTES • SERVES 8

Socca (also known as farinata) is a gluten-free flatbread made in the South of France and in Italy. I discovered it in my travels, and now we make it at home! The main ingredient is chickpea flour, making it high in protein and body-benefiting nutrients.

1 cup chickpea flour
1 teaspoon sea salt
½ teaspoon freshly ground black pepper
1 cup lukewarm filtered water
4 to 6 tablespoons extra virgin olive oil
2 teaspoons chopped fresh rosemary (optional)

1. Preheat the oven to 450°F.

2. Put a nonstick 12-inch pizza pan, cast-iron skillet, or traditional socca pan into the oven for 5 minutes.

3. While the pan is heating up, in a medium bowl, combine the chickpea flour with the salt and pepper. Slowly add the lukewarm water, whisking to eliminate any lumps.

4. Stir in 2 tablespoons of the olive oil and let sit while the oven heats. Your socca batter should be about the consistency of coconut milk.

5. Remove the pan from the oven, pour 2 tablespoons of the remaining olive oil into it, and swirl. Stir the rosemary into your socca batter, if using, and then immediately pour the batter into the pan. The batter should be spread very thin, like a crepe, for best results.

6. Bake for 10 to 15 minutes, until the socca is firm and the edges are set.

7. Remove the pan from the oven and preheat the broiler.

8. Brush the top of the socca with the remaining 1 to 2 tablespoons olive oil if it looks dry. Return to the top rack of the broiler and broil just long enough to brown it in spots.

9. Cut into wedges and serve hot or warm.

COOKED PLANT-BASED RECIPE

bomb hummus

PREP TIME: 9 MINUTES • TOTAL TIME: 9 MINUTES • SERVES 4 TO 8

This is based on a hummus recipe that my mom used to make, only with extra lemon, garlic, and fresh chives to crank the flavor way up! Hummus is the perfect protein-packed healthy dip for veggies, it's great in sandwiches and wraps, and it can even be used as a creamy salad dressing.

¼ cup lemon juice
1 tablespoon minced garlic
1 (15.5-ounce) can chickpeas, drained
1 bunch fresh chives
½ teaspoon sea salt
1 teaspoon ground cumin
¼ cup tahini
¼ cup extra virgin olive oil, plus more as needed
Sea salt and freshly ground black pepper to taste
Cayenne pepper or smoked paprika to taste (optional)

1. Combine all the ingredients except the salt, black pepper, and cayenne or paprika in a blender or food processor and blend until smooth, about 2 minutes.

2. Taste the hummus and add salt and black pepper as needed. I love to sprinkle in cayenne for a little kick or a bit of paprika for a roasted flavor.

3. If your hummus is too thick, add more olive oil or a little warm water and blend again.

4. Once you have your desired consistency, store in a glass container with an airtight lid in the fridge. The hummus will thicken as it chills.

PREDOMINANTLY LIVING PLANT-BASED RECIPE

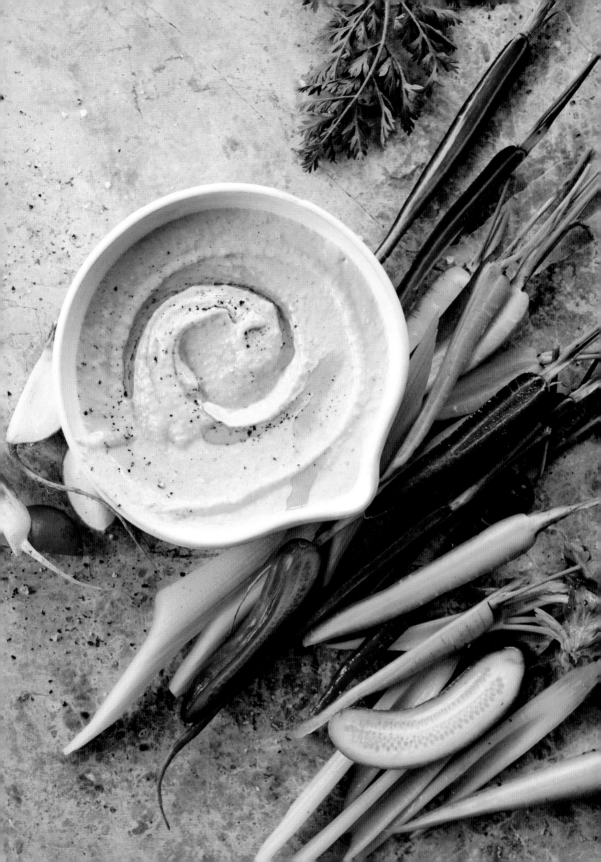

avo whip

PREP TIME: 4 MINUTES • TOTAL TIME: 4 MINUTES • SERVES 1 TO 4

This is a great topper for salads, it's also great in a sandwich, and I love it as a nourishing dip for raw veggies too!

1 ripe avocado
Sea salt and freshly ground black pepper
Juice of 1 lime

Place all the ingredients in a high-powered blender. Blend on high speed until smooth and creamy, about 1 minute, scraping the sides of the blender as needed. Store in an airtight container for a few days.

LIVING PLANT-BASED RECIPE

holy moly guacamole

PREP TIME: 12 MINUTES • TOTAL TIME: 12 MINUTES • SERVES 4 TO 6

Guacamole is arguably the most nutrient-dense condiment on the planet, full of heart-healthy fats, gut-friendly fiber, and blood pressure–regulating potassium. No taco is fully dressed without it if we're being perfectly honest! If you have never made it before, guac is super simple and there are a lot of ways to do it. This is my favorite.

2 medium ripe avocados, halved
½ cup finely chopped white onion
¼ cup finely chopped fresh cilantro
1 small jalapeño chile, seeds and ribs removed, finely chopped (optional)
1 tablespoon lime juice, plus more to taste
¼ teaspoon ground coriander
½ teaspoon sea salt, plus more to taste

1. Use a spoon to scoop the flesh out of the avocado and set the pit aside to use later (see Tip below). Cut out any bruised parts. Put the avocado flesh in a bowl and mash to the desired texture. I like my guacamole to have some texture, but if you like yours smooth, then just mix longer.

2. Add the onion, cilantro, jalapeño, if using, 1 tablespoon of lime juice, coriander, and ½ teaspoon of salt and mix to combine. Feel free to add more salt and lime juice to taste. The flavor of your guac is always best after it sits for a few minutes.

TIP: To keep your guac from going brown, put your saved pit in the middle of the bowl and drizzle the guac with extra lime or lemon juice before putting on an airtight lid. Your guacamole will keep in the fridge for up to 2 days, if you don't eat it all before that!

LIVING PLANT-BASED RECIPE

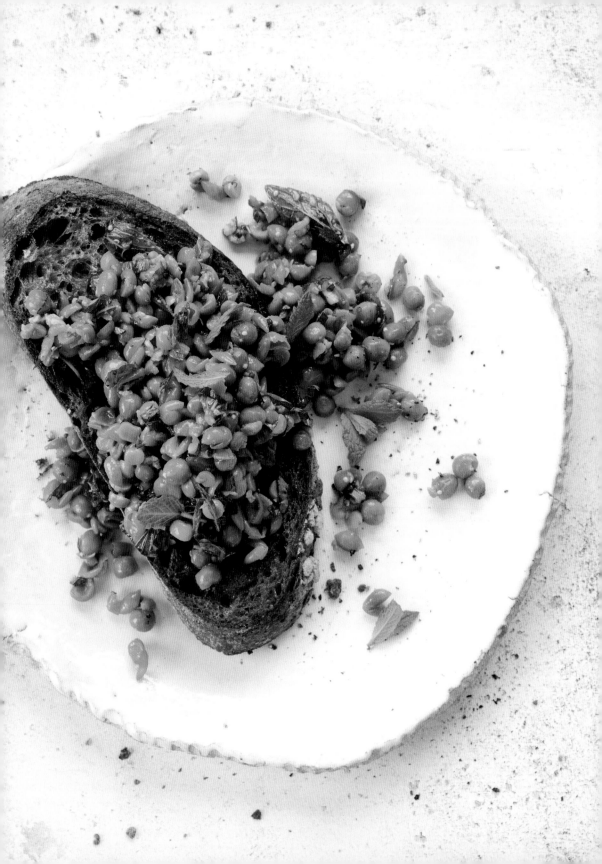

pea smash

PREP TIME: 18 MINUTES • TOTAL TIME: 18 MINUTES • SERVES 2 TO 4

If you're obsessed with avocado toast but looking for something that's a little different, try this! Pea smash is stealing the limelight from avocado with its delicious combination of garden peas, fresh mint, a bit of citrus, and a sprinkle of salt and pepper. This is a kid-friendly recipe that your whole family is sure to enjoy together on a slice of hearty toast or as a side dish or dip! A chef named Dave I met in Hossegor, France, was kind enough to share this recipe with me, and now I share it with you!

1 clove garlic, peeled
1 tablespoon extra virgin olive oil
1 teaspoon sea salt, plus more as needed
1 cup fresh or thawed frozen peas
½ teaspoon freshly ground black pepper
1 teaspoon lemon juice
1 teaspoon grainy mustard or another favorite mustard
¼ cup fresh mint leaves, shredded

1. Fill a medium pot with water and bring to a boil. Add the garlic, olive oil, and 1 teaspoon of salt and boil for 10 minutes, or until the garlic is soft.

2. Add the peas and boil for an additional 1 minute.

3. Drain the peas and garlic and place in a large bowl. Add the pepper, lemon juice, mustard, mint, and extra salt if needed.

4. Mix and mash with a fork until you achieve your desired consistency. For a smoother, spreadable consistency, transfer half of the mixture to a food processor and process until smooth, then mix it back in with the unblended mixture. Serve on toast, on top of a salad or rice cracker, or as a side dish with your meal.

PREDOMINANTLY LIVING PLANT-BASED RECIPE

pickled red onions

PREP TIME: 5 MINUTES • TOTAL TIME: 1 HOUR • SERVES 10

*Pickled red onions are
incredibly easy to make,
and they instantly take
just about any dish to
the next level! They also
support good digestion.
We always keep a jar
on hand to add to
sandwiches, avocado
toast, and salads.*

1 medium red onion
½ cup apple cider vinegar or white wine vinegar (my favorite)
1 tablespoon coconut sugar or maple syrup
1½ teaspoons sea salt
1 cup hot filtered water

1. Slice the red onion as thinly as possible (use a mandoline if you have one). Fill a mason jar with the red onion slices.

2. In a medium bowl, combine the vinegar, coconut sugar, salt, and hot water and stir until the sugar dissolves. This is your pickling mixture. Pour into the jar over the sliced onions, making sure they are immersed, and let sit for 1 hour. Cover and store in the fridge for up to 3 weeks.

LIVING PLANT-BASED RECIPE

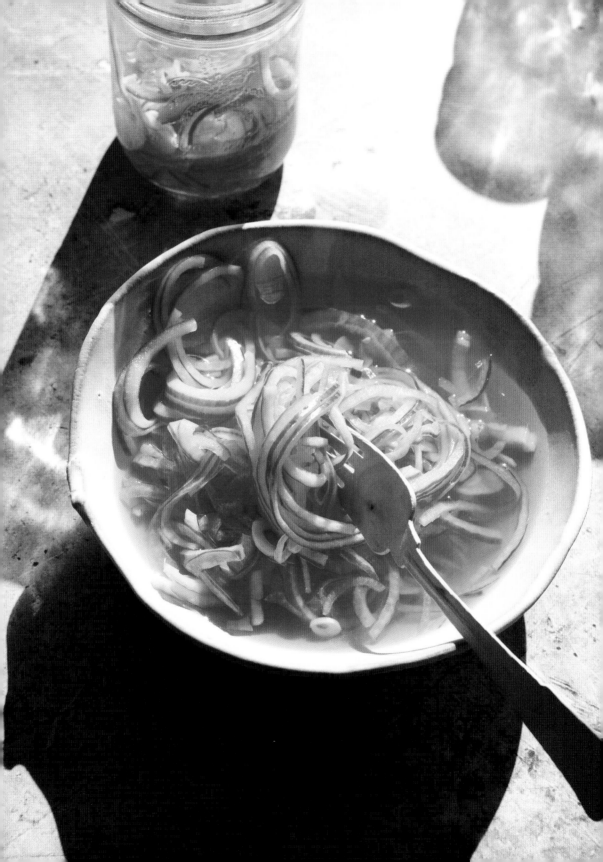

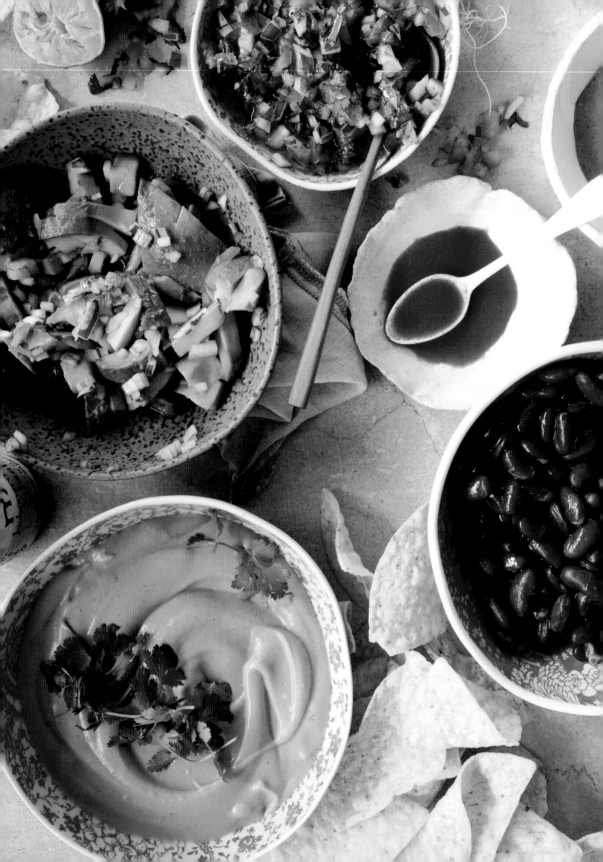

nach-yo everyday cheese sauce

PREP TIME: 10 MINUTES • TOTAL TIME: 30 MINUTES • SERVES 4 TO 8

This vegan cheese sauce is going to blow your mind and your taste buds! Use it as a dip for raw veggies or as a drizzle over steamed vegetables. Put it on rice, nachos, tacos, baked potatoes— whatever you like! This recipe is a favorite on my Instagram, and I hope it will become your favorite too!

2 cups peeled and chopped potato
1 cup chopped carrot
½ cup chopped yellow onion
3 cloves garlic, chopped
Extra virgin olive oil (optional)
½ cup raw cashews
½ cup nutritional yeast
1 teaspoon paprika
1 teaspoon sea salt, plus more as needed
Freshly ground black pepper
1 teaspoon hot sauce (optional)

1. In a large pot, combine the potato, carrot, onion, garlic, and a little water or olive oil, if using, and cook over medium-high heat for 10 minutes, then cover with an additional 2 cups hot water and simmer until the vegetables are soft, about 20 minutes.

2. Transfer everything from the pot into a food processor or blender. Add the cashews, nutritional yeast, paprika, 1 teaspoon of salt, and an additional ½ cup water.

3. Blend on high speed until the sauce is creamy and smooth, about 2 minutes.

4. Season with black pepper and add the hot sauce, if using, and a little more salt if needed. Store in an airtight container in the refrigerator for up to 1 week.

COOKED PLANT-BASED RECIPE

macadamia nut pesto

PREP TIME: 9 MINUTES • TOTAL TIME: 10 MINUTES • SERVES 4 TO 6

Macadamias are the nut of Hawaii, and this pesto is going to dress up your pasta with an island twist!

1 cup macadamia nuts
2 cups fresh basil leaves
2 cloves garlic, peeled
Juice of 1 lemon
¼ cup extra virgin olive oil
½ teaspoon sea salt
Freshly ground black pepper

1. Toast the macadamia nuts in a small skillet over medium heat, tossing constantly until golden, about 3 minutes. Remove from the skillet and let the nuts cool a little.

2. Put the macadamia nuts, basil, garlic, and half of the lemon juice into a food processor and process on high speed, slowly adding the oil through the hole in the lid, until creamy.

3. Add the salt, season with pepper, and add the remaining lemon juice. Store in an airtight container in the fridge for up to 1 week.

LIVING PLANT-BASED RECIPE

avocado ceviche

PREP TIME: 14 MINUTES • TOTAL TIME: 14 MINUTES • SERVES 2

This vegan take on ceviche, using avocados instead of fish, is one of our favorite sides to whip up and enjoy on top of a salad, with potato crisps, or wrapped up in lettuce cups or pita.

1 celery stalk
1 small cucumber
1 small red bell pepper
½ red onion
1 avocado
¼ cup chopped fresh basil leaves
¼ cup chopped fresh cilantro leaves (optional)
¼ cup lemon juice
Sea salt and freshly ground black pepper

1. Chop the celery, cucumber, bell pepper, and red onion into small bite-sized cubes.

2. Chop the avocado into bite-sized cubes as well and mix with the chopped vegetables. Stir in the basil and cilantro, if using.

3. Add the lemon juice and season with salt and pepper.

LIVING PLANT-BASED RECIPE

everyday og salad dressing

PREP TIME: 4 MINUTES • TOTAL TIME: 4 MINUTES • MAKES ABOUT ½ CUP

This is a go-to for green salads and Earth Bowls. It's quick, simple, and crowd-pleasing, and it accentuates the flavors of the nourishing star ingredients in your dish without overdoing things. Once you learn to make this dressing, you'll never want to purchase another store-bought, processed salad dressing again!

⅓ cup extra virgin olive oil
1 tablespoon lemon juice
2 tablespoons maple syrup
2 teaspoons Dijon or stone-ground mustard
½ teaspoon garlic powder (optional)
Sea salt and freshly ground black pepper

Combine all the ingredients in a mason jar and seal tightly with a lid. Shake to mix well. Store in the fridge for up to 1 week.

PREDOMINANTLY LIVING PLANT-BASED RECIPE

caesar dressing

PREP TIME: 4 MINUTES • TOTAL TIME: 4 MINUTES • MAKES ¾ CUP TO 1 CUP

One of the quickest ways to ruin a salad is by drenching it in a dressing that is full of sugar and processed ingredients. This natural, vegan Caesar dressing packs all the flavor of traditional Caesar without any additives to weigh you down!

½ cup raw cashews, soaked overnight
½ cup filtered water
1 tablespoon extra virgin olive oil
2 tablespoons fresh lemon juice
1 tablespoon Dijon mustard
1 teaspoon garlic powder, or more if you like it strong
½ tablespoon vegan Worcestershire sauce (I use Wizard's gluten-free brand)
2 teaspoons capers
½ teaspoon fine grain sea salt and pepper, or to taste

Place all the ingredients in a high-powered blender and blend for 1 minute on high until smooth and creamy.

PREDOMINANTLY LIVING PLANT-BASED RECIPE

vegan aioli

PREP TIME: 10 MINUTES • TOTAL TIME: 13 MINUTES • MAKES ABOUT ½ CUP

Aioli sounds fancy, but it takes only a few minutes to make and it's the perfect base for creating a wide range of vegan-friendly dips and spreads. Once you have your aioli base, you can add a variety of fresh herbs and spices to make it your own with a bold flavor that makes vegan anything but boring!

½ cup raw cashews
½ cup filtered water
Pinch sea salt and freshly ground black pepper
Optional add-ins: minced fresh dill, basil, and/or garlic, lemon juice, and red pepper flakes

1. Place the cashews, water, salt, and pepper in a high-powered blender. Blend on high speed until creamy. This is your aioli base.

2. Add whichever flavorful add-ins you like.

3. Store in an airtight glass jar in the fridge for up to 1 week.

NOTE: *If you're not using a high-powered blender, adding a drizzle of olive oil or a little extra water will help emulsify the dressing.*

PREDOMINANTLY LIVING PLANT-BASED RECIPE

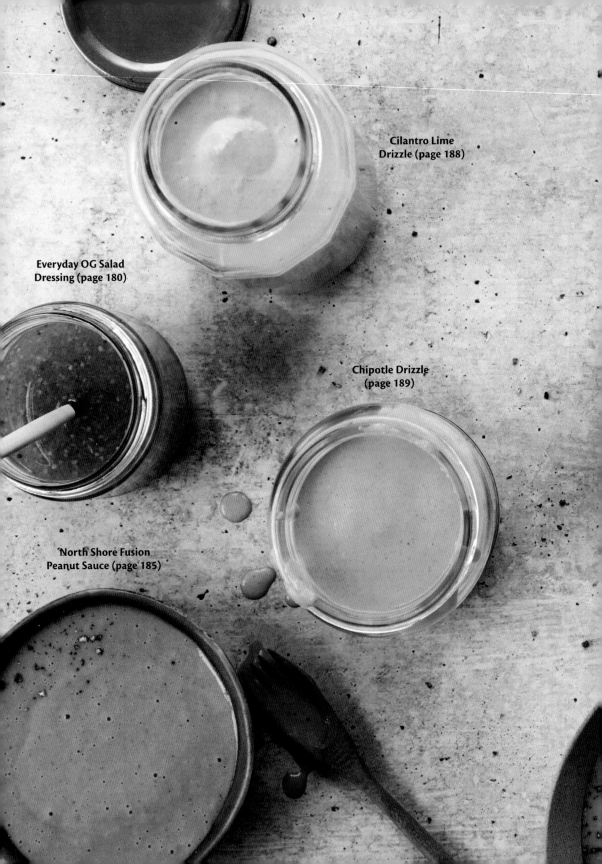

Cilantro Lime
Drizzle (page 188)

Everyday OG Salad
Dressing (page 180)

Chipotle Drizzle
(page 189)

North Shore Fusion
Peanut Sauce (page 185)

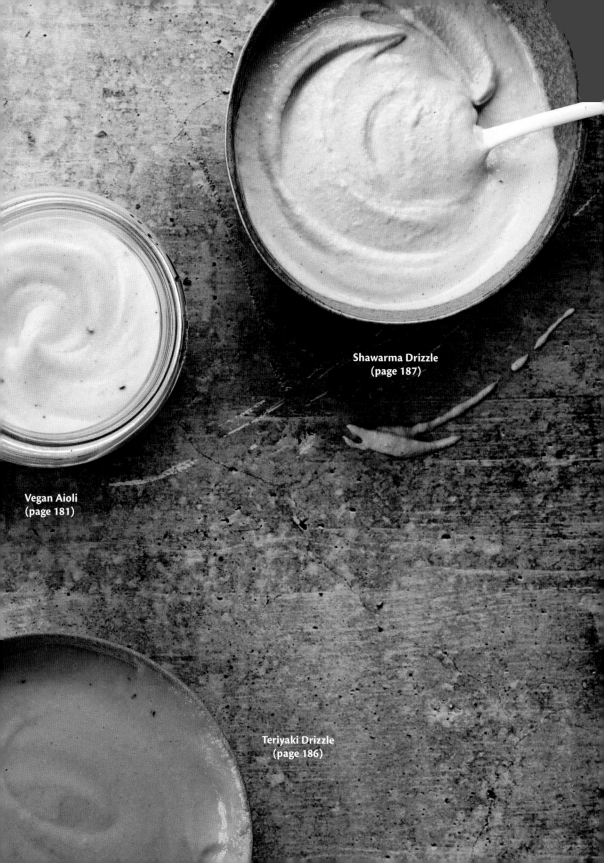

Shawarma Drizzle
(page 187)

Vegan Aioli
(page 181)

Teriyaki Drizzle
(page 186)

vegan sour cream

PREP TIME: 10 MINUTES • TOTAL TIME: 13 MINUTES • MAKES ABOUT 1 CUP

It's easier than you may think to make a thick, creamy plant-based sour cream! If you're steering clear of dairy, this is your ideal swap.

1 cup raw cashews
½ cup filtered water
1½ tablespoons lemon juice, plus more if desired
1 teaspoon apple cider vinegar
½ teaspoon fine sea salt
½ teaspoon Dijon mustard

1. Place all the ingredients in a high-powered blender. Blend on high speed until creamy.

2. Store in an airtight glass jar in the fridge for up to 1 week.

NOTES: *If you're not using a high-powered blender, add a little extra water for a smooth and creamy consistency. I love this sour cream with my Lemon Pepper Potato Fries (page 160), Chipotle Lime Black Bean Bowl (page 114), and Beach Bum Chili (page 144).*

PREDOMINANTLY LIVING PLANT-BASED RECIPE

north shore fusion peanut sauce

PREP TIME: 12 MINUTES • TOTAL TIME: 25 MINUTES • MAKES ABOUT 3 CUPS

I originally created this sauce for my summer rolls, but I've found that it's perfect for drizzling over rice, stir-fried veggies, and nourishing salad bowls too! If you are allergic to peanuts, try swapping the peanut butter in this recipe for cashew butter or tahini.

1 (14-ounce) can unsweetened coconut milk (full-fat for better consistency and full flavor)
¼ cup Thai red curry paste
¾ cup natural creamy peanut butter (or ¾ cup cashew butter or tahini)
½ teaspoon sea salt
¾ cup packed coconut sugar
2 tablespoons apple cider vinegar or white wine vinegar
½ cup filtered water

1. Combine all the ingredients in a medium saucepan. Place over medium heat and bring to a gentle boil, whisking constantly.

2. Reduce the heat to low and simmer for 3 to 5 minutes. Remove from the heat and allow the sauce to cool and thicken.

3. Use immediately, or store in an airtight glass jar in the refrigerator for up to 2 weeks. The sauce will thicken in the fridge, so you may need to add a little water before serving.

COOKED PLANT-BASED RECIPE

teriyaki drizzle

PREP TIME: 3 MINUTES • TOTAL TIME: 3 MINUTES • MAKES ABOUT ¾ CUP

Who doesn't love the sweet, sour, salty, and savory flavor combo of teriyaki? This is a dream sauce for drizzling over rice, stir-fries, or over my Teri Poke Bowl (page 113).

½ cup raw cashews
½ cup filtered water
1 tablespoon gluten-free teriyaki sauce, plus more as needed
Sea salt and freshly ground black pepper

1. Place the cashews, water, and 1 tablespoon of teriyaki sauce in a high-powered blender or food processor. Blend until smooth and creamy.

2. Season with salt and pepper. Some teriyaki sauces are stronger than others, so feel free to up the amount of teriyaki as desired!

3. Store in an airtight glass jar in the fridge for up to 1 week.

PREDOMINANTLY LIVING PLANT-BASED RECIPE

shawarma drizzle

PREP TIME: 10 MINUTES • TOTAL TIME: 14 MINUTES • MAKES ABOUT ¾ CUP

With the flavor combo of freshly squeezed lemon juice, parsley, mint, and garlic, you're going to have to make a rule for yourself: Repeat after me, do not eat straight from the jar! But if you do, no judgment here. This sauce is just that good.

½ cup raw cashews
½ cup filtered water
2 tablespoons lemon juice
2 tablespoons fresh parsley leaves
2 tablespoons fresh mint leaves
1 clove garlic, peeled
Sea salt and freshly ground pepper to taste

1. Place all the ingredients in a high-powered blender. Blend on high speed until creamy.

2. Store in an airtight glass jar in the fridge for up to 1 week.

NOTE: *If you're not using a high-powered blender, add a little extra water to get to a smooth consistency. You can also swap out the parsley or mint for dill, if you prefer.*

LIVING PLANT-BASED RECIPE

cilantro lime drizzle

This delicious drizzle ties a whole meal together! It's a classic pairing with Mexican dishes like tacos, burritos, and rice and beans, or on top of a big Earth Bowl or salad.

½ cup raw cashews
½ cup filtered water
½ cup fresh cilantro leaves
1 tablespoon lime or lemon juice
¼ teaspoon freshly ground black pepper
¼ teaspoon sea salt
¼ ground cumin (optional)
Dash of your favorite hot sauce (optional)

1. Place all the ingredients in a high-powered blender. Blend together on high until creamy.
2. Store in an airtight glass jar in the fridge for up to 1 week.

NOTE: *If you're not using a high-powered blender, add a little extra water to get to a smooth consistency.*

LIVING PLANT-BASED RECIPE

chipotle drizzle

This is another sauce that's great on tacos, burritos, and salads for next-level flavor. I used to make this with yogurt before going vegan, but I discovered that creamy blended cashews are a perfect alternative to dairy that won't irritate your digestive system.

½ cup raw cashews
½ cup filtered water
1½ tablespoons nutritional yeast
1 teaspoon chipotle chile powder
1 clove garlic or ¼ teaspoon garlic powder
1 teaspoon smoked paprika
1 tablespoon lemon juice
2 teaspoons maple syrup
Pinch cayenne pepper (optional)
Sea salt to taste

1. Place all the ingredients in a high-powered blender. Blend on high speed until creamy. Add more water if needed for desired thickness and adjust the seasonings to taste.

2. Store in an airtight glass jar in the fridge for up to 1 week.

NOTE: *If you're not using a high-powered blender, add a little extra water to get to a smooth consistency.*

PREDOMINANTLY LIVING PLANT-BASED RECIPE

hawaiian mactella

PREP TIME: 3 MINUTES • TOTAL TIME: 4 MINUTES • MAKES ABOUT 2 CUPS

Store-bought Nutella is amazing, no argument there. But some of the ingredients, like palm oil and processed sugar, are less than healthy, which is where this homemade version comes in. I've replaced the traditional hazelnuts with macadamias for a Hawaiian spin.

3 cups raw unsalted macadamia nuts
1 cup vegan chocolate chips

1. Place the macadamia nuts in a high-powered blender or food processor. Blend on high speed until you have smooth macadamia nut butter, about 1 minute.
2. Melt the chocolate in a small saucepan over low heat, stirring frequently and being careful not to let it burn.
3. Remove the chocolate from the heat and stir in the macadamia butter.
4. Transfer to an airtight glass jar and store in the fridge for up to 1 week.

PREDOMINANTLY LIVING PLANT-BASED RECIPE

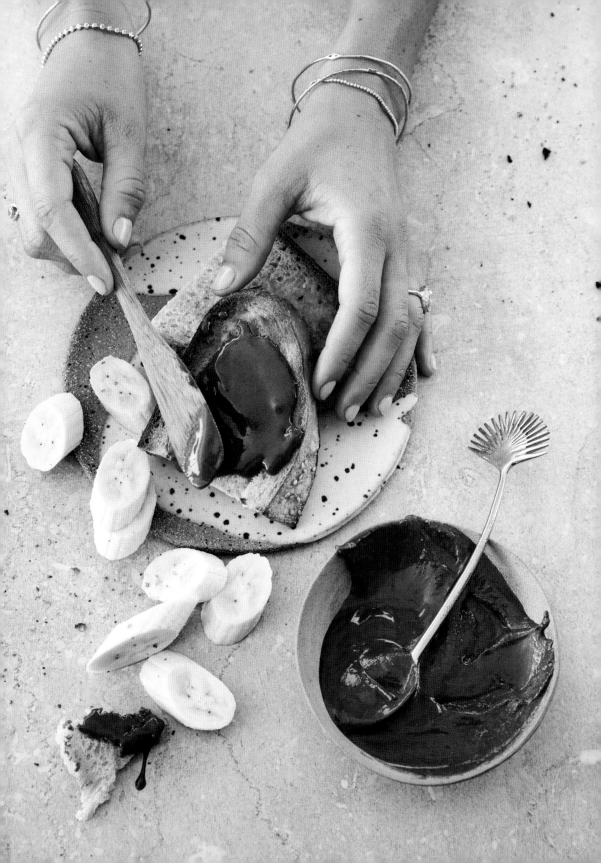

salted coconut caramel sauce

PREP TIME: 32 MINUTES • TOTAL TIME: 35 MINUTES • MAKES ABOUT 2 CUPS

This insanely delicious vegan caramel sauce is great for drizzling on smoothie bowls, on vegan ice cream, or on fresh fruit. Isn't it amazing what you do with coconuts?

2 cups packed coconut sugar
2 cups full-fat canned unsweetened coconut milk
½ teaspoon sea salt

1. Combine all the ingredients in a medium saucepan. Place over medium heat and cook, stirring constantly, as the mixture comes to a boil and the sauce reduces and takes on a thick consistency, 35 to 45 minutes.

2. Test the consistency of the caramel by spooning a few drops from your saucepan into a cup of ice-cold water once you're around the 35-minute mark. If soft balls form when you pick up the caramel and drop it between your fingers, you know the caramel is done. If it is not done, try again after boiling for another 3 to 5 minutes.

3. Pour the caramel sauce into a glass jar, cool completely, cover, and store in the fridge for up to 1 week.

PREDOMINANTLY LIVING
PLANT-BASED RECIPE

vegan chocolate sauce

PREP TIME: 22 MINUTES • TOTAL TIME: 42 MINUTES • MAKES ABOUT 2 CUPS

This all-natural, 100 percent plant-based chocolate sauce is perfect for topping vegan ice cream or for having a chocolate fondue party!

1 (14-ounce) can full-fat unsweetened coconut milk
½ cup packed coconut sugar
⅓ cup unsweetened cacao powder
2 tablespoons coconut butter or coconut oil
Seeds from 1 vanilla bean or 1 teaspoon pure vanilla extract
Pinch sea salt

1. In a small saucepan over medium heat, whisk together the coconut milk, coconut sugar, and cacao powder until smooth.

2. Reduce the heat to low and simmer, stirring, for 10 minutes. Remove from the heat and stir in the coconut butter or coconut oil, vanilla, and salt.

3. Allow the sauce to cool for 20 minutes before storing in the fridge for up to 2 weeks.

COOKED PLANT-BASED RECIPE

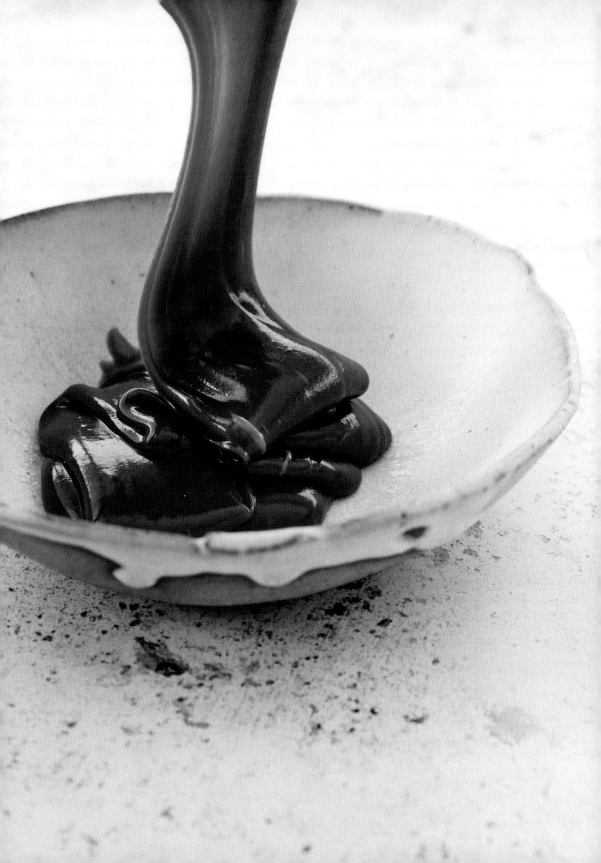

plant over processed snacks

It is all too easy to tear into a bag of chips or a candy bar when you're hungry. Processed treats are tasty, and they can seem like a good idea in the moment. But remember our mantra: Plant Over Processed. With some preparation and planning, you can make better choices by having these healthy and delicious snacks at the ready.

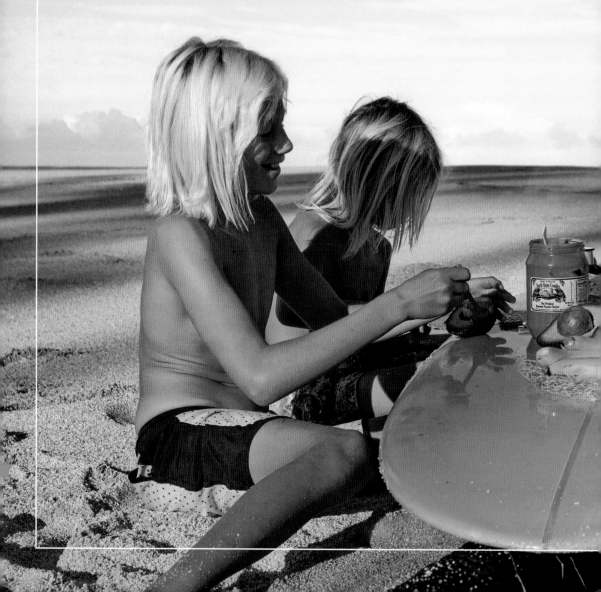

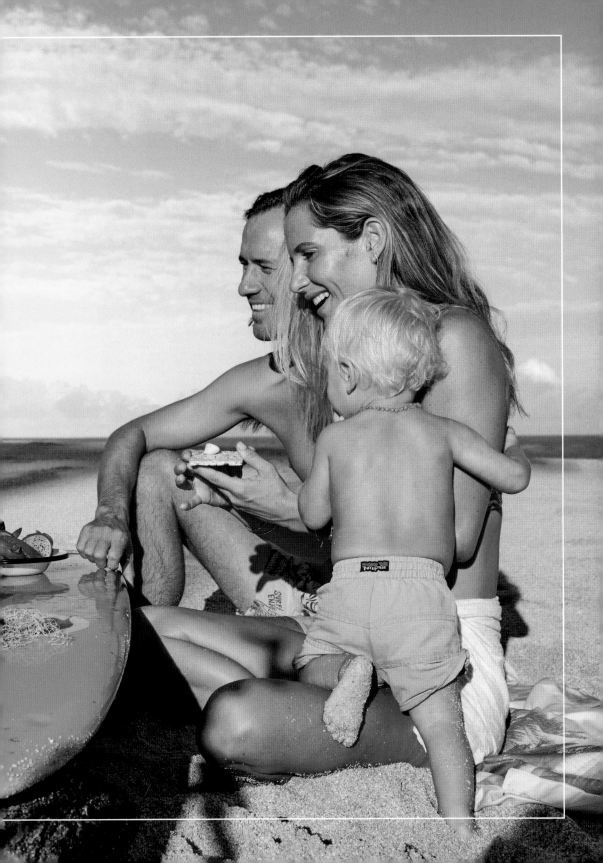

peanut butter banana toasties

PREP TIME: 3 MINUTES • TOTAL TIME: 3 MINUTES • SERVES 4

This is one of our favorite snacks to bring to the beach, deconstructed, and build on top of a makeshift beach table, aka a surfboard! All you need is your favorite nut butter, some rice cakes or corn cakes, and a few banana slices.

4 tablespoons natural peanut butter
4 rice cakes or corn cakes
2 bananas, peeled and sliced

Spread the peanut butter on the rice cakes or corn cakes and top with the banana slices.

TIP: *If you're feeling "extra," add a sprinkle of coconut sugar, a dash of cinnamon, and a drizzle of maple syrup. Yum!*

PREDOMINANTLY LIVING PLANT-BASED RECIPE

avocado toasties

PREP TIME: 3 MINUTES • TOTAL TIME: 3 MINUTES • SERVES 4

This is a great swap if you are gluten-intolerant and feel like you're missing out on the avocado toast craze. And if you love your avo toast but are trying to cut back on bread, this will be your jam too!

1 ripe avocado, halved and pitted
4 rice cakes or corn cakes
Sea salt and freshly ground black pepper
Lemon or lime juice
Pickled Red Onions (page 174; optional)

1. Peel and slice the avocado. Top the rice cakes or corn cakes with the avo slices, or mash up the avocado and spread it on.
2. Sprinkle with salt and pepper, then drizzle with lemon or lime juice. And if you want to get fancy, add a few slices of pickled red onion!

PREDOMINANTLY LIVING PLANT-BASED RECIPE

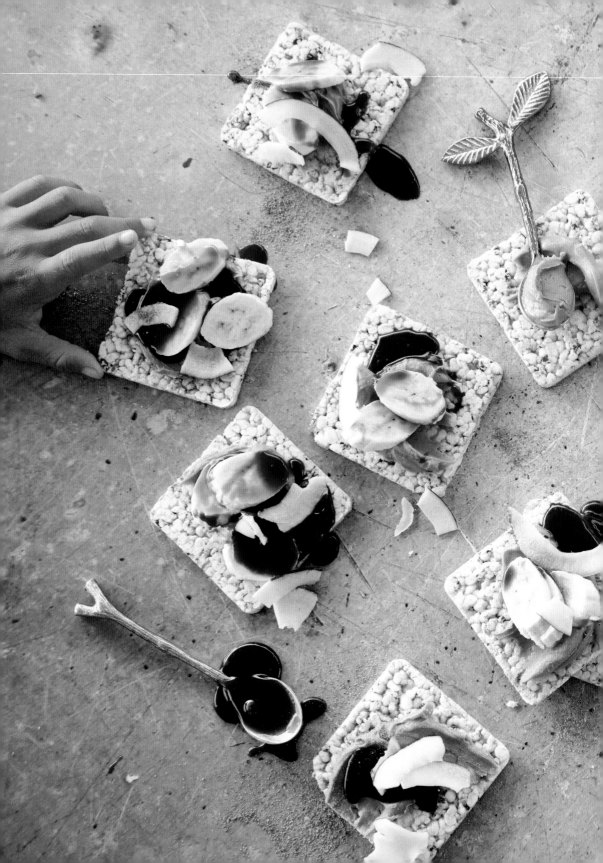

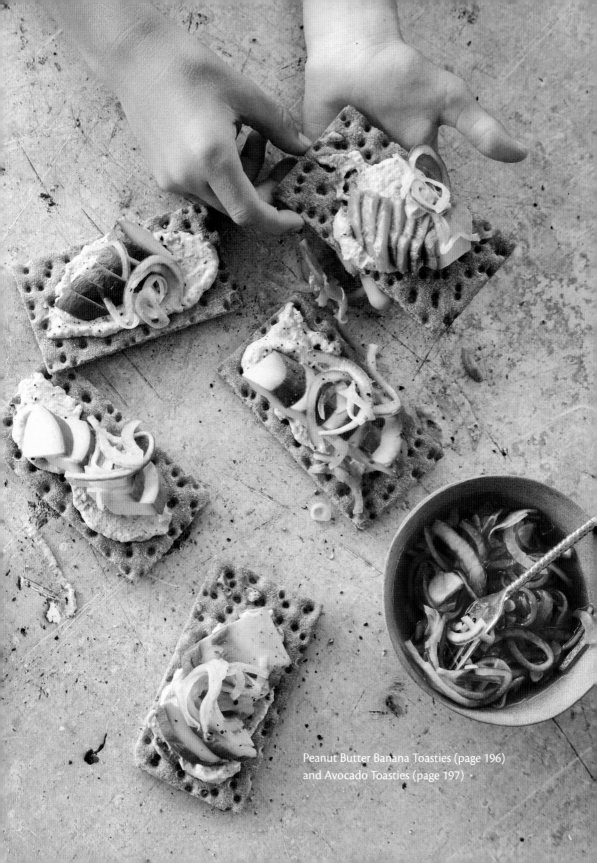

Peanut Butter Banana Toasties (page 196)
and Avocado Toasties (page 197) ·

blue crush slush

This one sounds a little weird, but it is delicious! The frozen blueberries turn the oat milk blue and the granola makes it feel like you are biting into a slushy blueberry muffin! Add dried blueberries or dried mango pieces for chew, and a drizzle of extra sweetness if you must!

2 cups frozen blueberries
1 ripe banana, sliced
½ cup granola
1 cup oat milk or other favorite nut milk

Mix the blueberries, banana, and granola in a cereal bowl or two. Pour over the oat or nut milk and let the frozen berries make everything slushy!

PREDOMINANTLY LIVING PLANT-BASED RECIPE

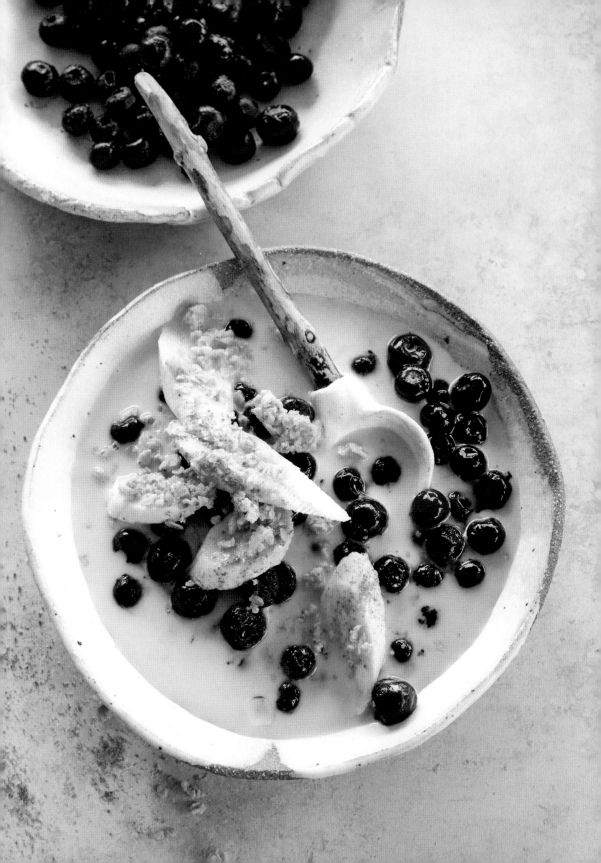

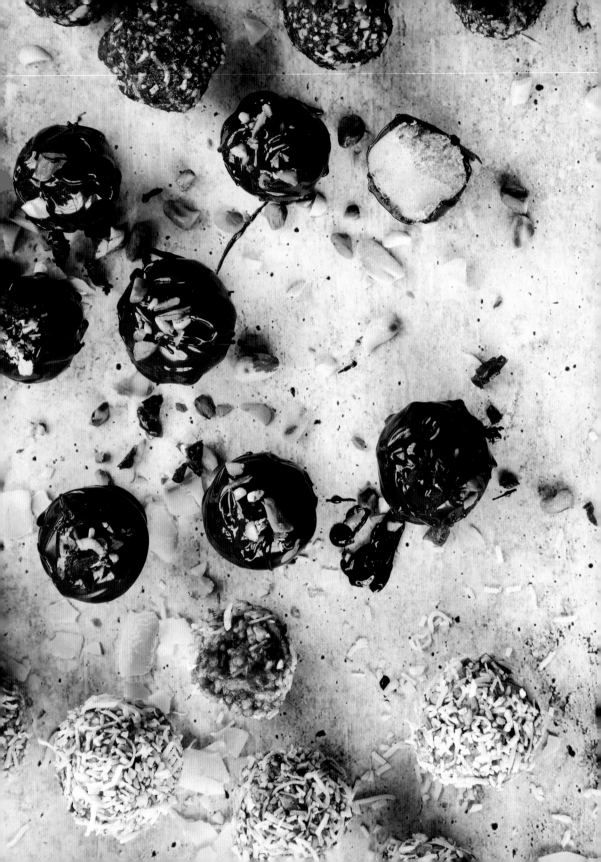

chocolate energy balls

PREP TIME: 30 MINUTES • TOTAL TIME: 30 MINUTES • MAKES 20 BALLS

These Chocolate Energy Balls are healthy, I swear, but they sure do taste like dessert! If you have a sweet tooth like I do, having healthy, bite-sized sweet treats on hand is essential for sticking to your health goals.

2 cups hazelnuts
2 cups pitted dates (Medjool are best, but Deglet Noor are good too)
2 tablespoons cacao powder
2 teaspoons vanilla bean paste or 1 teaspoon pure vanilla extract
¼ cup finely shredded unsweetened coconut, plus 1 to 2 cups extra for rolling

1. Preheat the oven to 350°F.

2. Spread the hazelnuts on a baking sheet and toast in the oven for 10 to 15 minutes, until fragrant. Remove from the oven and roll the toasted hazelnuts in a kitchen towel to remove some of the skins.

3. Put the dates, cacao powder, and vanilla in a food processor and process until well combined and the consistency of a thick paste. Add the hazelnuts and the ¼ cup shredded coconut and pulse until well combined. Transfer from the food processor to a large bowl. Spread the extra shredded coconut on a plate for rolling. With dampened hands, roll the mixture into 20 1-inch balls, then roll each ball in the extra shredded coconut to coat.

4. Store in an airtight container in the fridge for up to 3 weeks, or in the freezer for up to 3 months.

PREDOMINANTLY LIVING PLANT-BASED RECIPE

salted caramel coconut energy balls

PREP TIME: 30 MINUTES • TOTAL TIME: 35 MINUTES • MAKES 20 BALLS

This recipe is a twist on a treat that my mom used to make for us every Christmas. These caramel coconut balls traditionally call for a lot of butter and brown sugar, but I've found that if I use a bit of coconut oil and a small amount of coconut sugar instead, they are just as good. It's a win-win! These were an absolute saving grace when I changed my diet, satisfying my sweet tooth and keeping me on the road to health. You may want to double this recipe—they go quickly!

3 cups pitted Medjool dates
3 tablespoons filtered water
1 cup packed coconut sugar
2 tablespoons coconut oil
1 teaspoon pure vanilla extract
4 cups organic crispy rice cereal (not puffed rice because it will affect the texture)
½ cup shredded unsweetened coconut, plus 1 to 2 cups extra for rolling
½ teaspoon sea salt

1. Mince the dates into small pieces, until sticky. Add the water, coconut sugar, coconut oil, and minced dates to a large skillet. Stir constantly over medium-low heat until you have a paste and see small bubbles, about 10 minutes.

2. Stir in the vanilla and remove from the heat. Transfer the date mixture to a large bowl and set aside until it is cool enough to handle but still warm enough to mix and roll easily.

3. Fold in the crispy rice cereal, the ½ cup shredded coconut, and salt. Spread the extra shredded coconut on a plate for rolling.

4. With dampened hands, roll the mixture into 20 1-inch balls, then roll each one in the extra coconut to coat.

5. Store in an airtight container in the refrigerator for up to 3 weeks, or in the freezer for up to 3 months.

COOKED PLANT-BASED RECIPE

buckeye protein balls

This is another version of a recipe that I had been eating for years. The original has loads of butter and refined sugar in it. I completely revamped it to be vegan and nourishing, and still delicious! This simple four-ingredient recipe can be made with your favorite vegan protein powder.

2½ cups natural peanut butter
¾ cup vanilla plant protein powder
⅓ cup maple syrup
Pinch sea salt (optional)
2 cups vegan chocolate chips

1. Mix together the peanut butter, protein powder, maple syrup, and salt, if using, in a large bowl. With dampened hands, roll into 10 bite-sized balls.

2. Melt the chocolate chips in a small saucepan on the stovetop over low heat. Or microwave in a microwave-safe bowl on high for 30 seconds, stir, microwave for an additional 30 seconds, and stir again to fully melt.

3. Poke a chopstick into each ball, then dip them into the melted chocolate until thoroughly coated.

4. Place the balls on a plate and put in the fridge to cool and set for 1 hour.

5. Transfer to an airtight container and store in the fridge for up to 2 weeks.

PREDOMINANTLY LIVING PLANT-BASED RECIPE

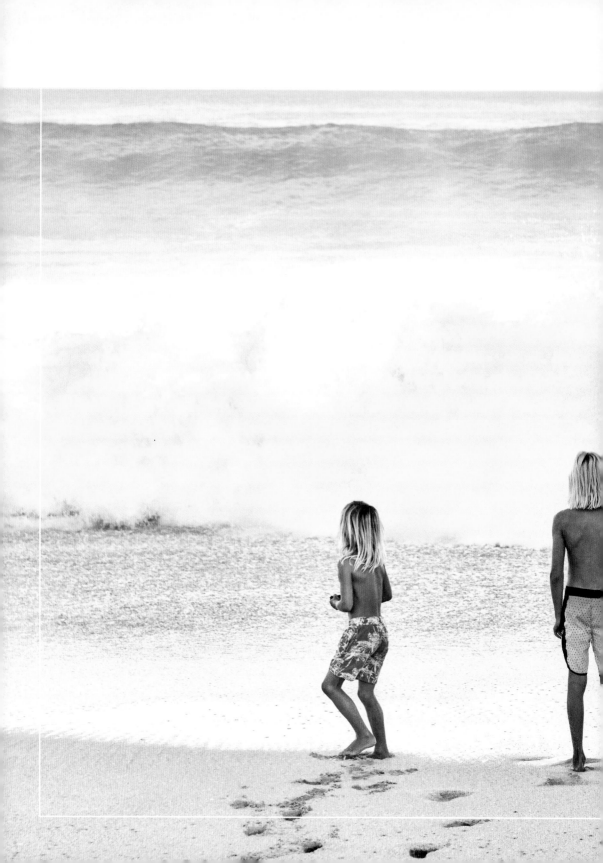

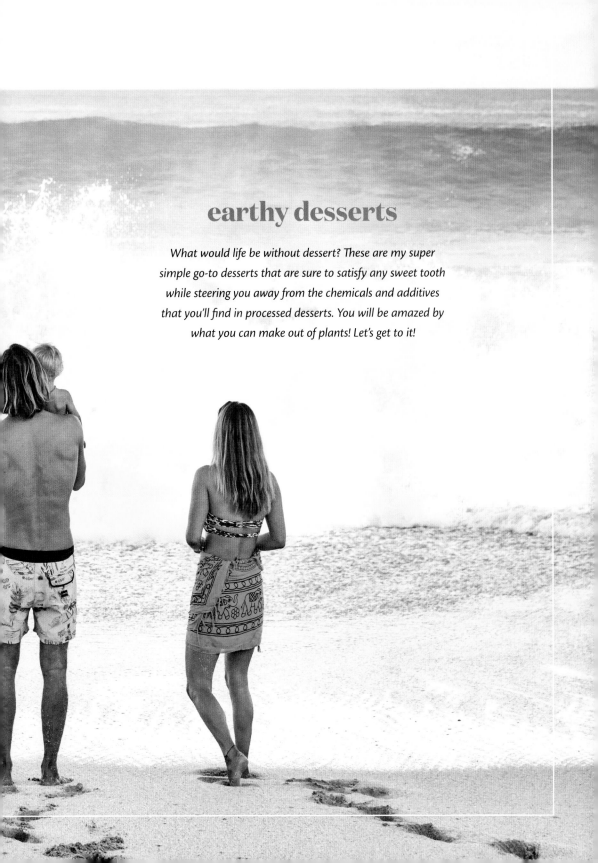

earthy desserts

What would life be without dessert? These are my super simple go-to desserts that are sure to satisfy any sweet tooth while steering you away from the chemicals and additives that you'll find in processed desserts. You will be amazed by what you can make out of plants! Let's get to it!

cookies 'n cream vanilla ice cream

PREP TIME: 15 MINUTES • TOTAL TIME: 15 MINUTES + 2 HOURS • SERVES 6

What if I were to tell you that you can give your kids bananas in the form of ice cream and they wouldn't know the difference? This is so fun to make and even more fun to eat! No need to worry about tummy aches from dairy and processed sugars when you can make something just as delicious using wholesome ingredients.

FOR THE COOKIE DOUGH:

3 tablespoons vegan butter or coconut oil
½ cup natural peanut butter
½ cup packed coconut sugar
1 teaspoon pure vanilla extract
¾ cup all-purpose gluten-free flour
¼ cup vegan chocolate chunks
1 to 2 tablespoons oat milk

FOR THE ICE CREAM BASE:

6 frozen ripe bananas, sliced
¼ cup plant milk
1 teaspoon pure vanilla extract
1 scoop vanilla plant protein powder (optional)

1. To make the cookie dough, mix all the ingredients together in a large bowl until well combined.

2. Wrap in wax paper and store in an airtight container in the freezer.

3. To make the ice cream base, place all the ingredients in a high-powered blender. Blend until thick and creamy and ice cream–like.

4. Take half of the cookie dough mixture and roughly chop it (freeze the rest for up to 3 months).

5. Tip the contents of the blender into a large bowl or container and fold through the chopped cookie dough, leaving some extra to decorate the top.

6. Cover and place back in the freezer for an extra hour or two for added thickness.

NOTE: *If you're not using a high-powered blender, add extra milk in the ice cream base to get to a smooth consistency.*

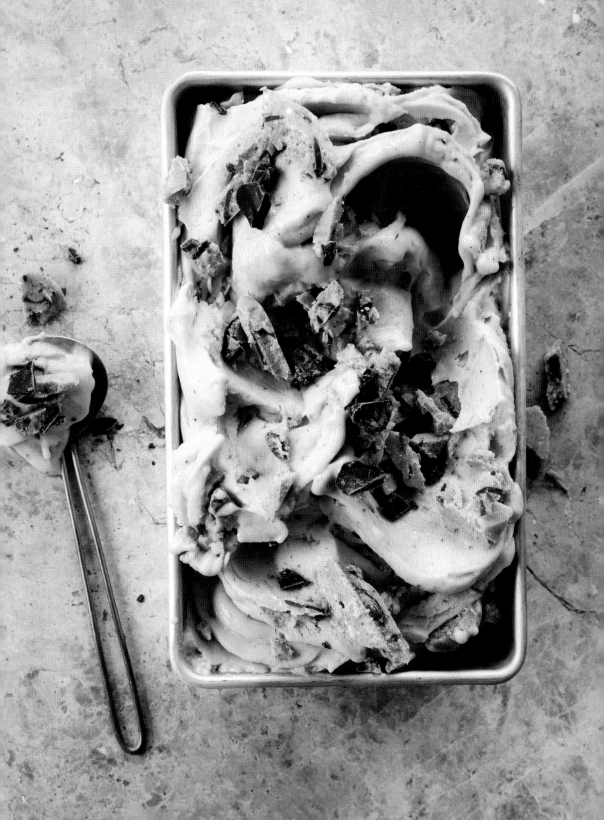

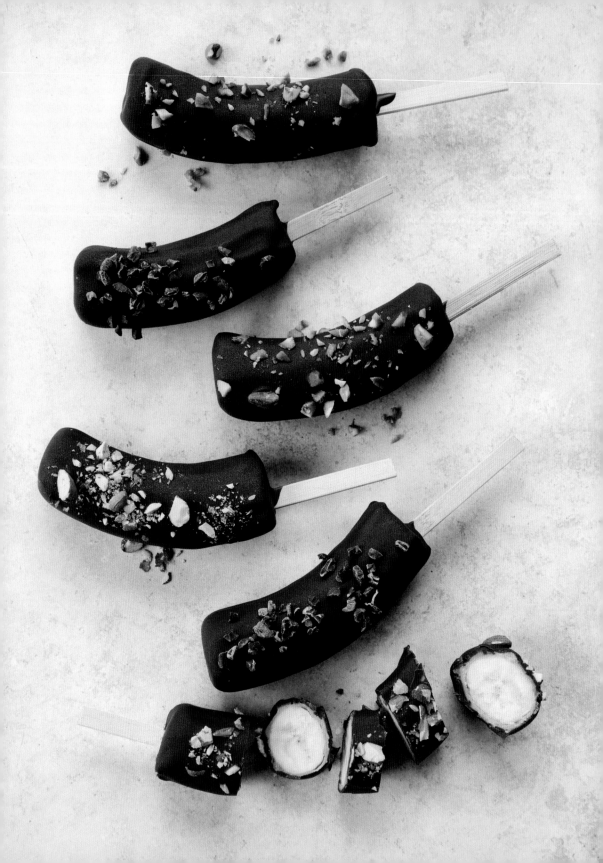

frozen chocolate peanut butter banana bites

PREP TIME: 5 MINUTES • TOTAL TIME: 5 MINUTES + 3 HOURS • SERVES 3

Frozen bananas taste like sweet ice cream! You can prepare this dish as chocolate-dipped ice pops or as bite-sized treats. Both ways are insanely delicious. Dress these up with cacao nibs or crushed peanuts. This one looks fancy, but it's actually super easy to create at home.

3 ripe bananas
½ cup smooth natural peanut butter
½ cup vegan chocolate chips
Toppings: cacao nibs and/or crushed peanuts (optional)

1. Peel each banana and stick a wooden ice pop stick or chopstick into one end. Place the bananas on a wax paper–covered plate and put them in the freezer for at least 2 hours.

2. Meanwhile, microwave the peanut butter in a deep cup until softened and slightly warmed. Dip the frozen bananas into the warm peanut butter to coat, then place back in the freezer for 30 minutes to harden.

3. Melt the chocolate chips in another deep cup and dip the peanut butter–coated bananas into the melted chocolate, giving them a second coat. Sprinkle on any desired toppings before the chocolate hardens. Place back in the freezer for 30 minutes to harden before eating.

PREDOMINANTLY LIVING PLANT-BASED RECIPE

caramel chewies

Dates are nature's candy, full of vitamins, minerals, and fiber! I love them for baking, smoothies, and just on their own. But more than anything, I love them in these decadent, all-natural Caramel Chewies!

12 Medjool dates
¼ cup natural peanut butter or almond butter
¼ cup vegan chocolate chips
¼ cup crushed peanuts or slivered almonds (optional)
Sea salt for sprinkling

1. Slice each date open enough to remove the pit. Fill each date with 1 teaspoon of the peanut butter or almond butter. Arrange the dates on a baking sheet or plate.
2. In a microwave-safe bowl, melt the chocolate chips for 30 seconds to 1 minute, stir to create a smooth chocolate sauce, and drizzle over each date.
3. Sprinkle each date with the crushed peanuts or slivered almonds, if using, and a tiny bit of salt.
4. Freeze the dates for at least 1 hour for the best texture before serving. The dates can be stored in an airtight container in the freezer for up to 30 days.

PREDOMINANTLY LIVING PLANT-BASED RECIPE

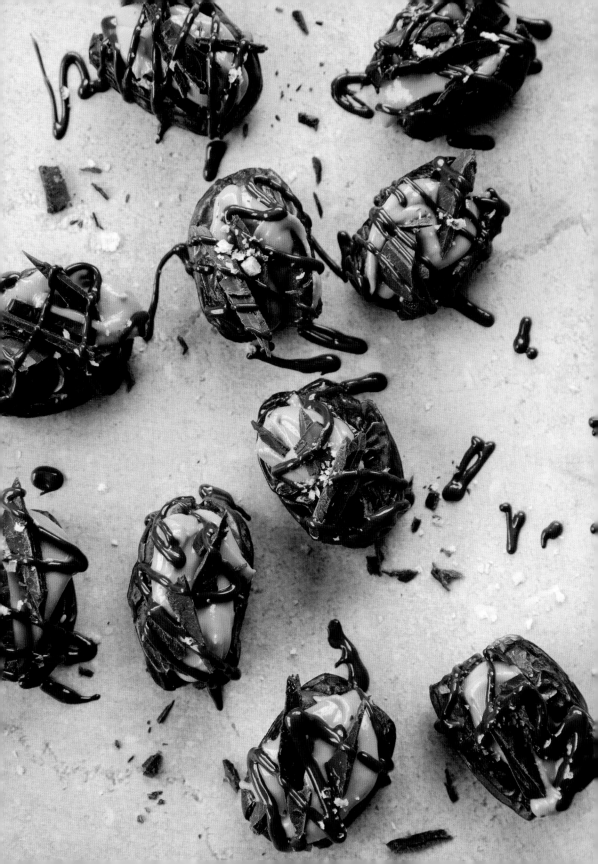

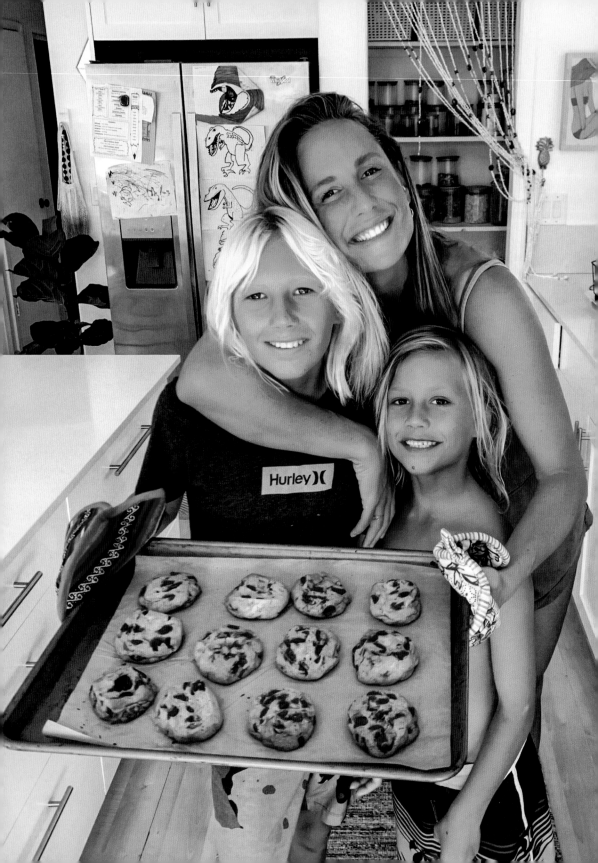

magic cookies

PREP TIME: 10 MINUTES • TOTAL TIME: 30 MINUTES • SERVES 2

Have you ever made cookies out of chickpeas? Is your first thought "Ew"? I challenge you to make this and see for yourself why these are called magic cookies! They taste insanely good, but are naturally gluten-free, dairy-free, vegan, and full of protein, fiber, and minerals. Feel free to make these into brownies or in little muffin tins. This recipe has been tried thousands of times by people all around the world, and I get the same response every time: It's hard to believe a cookie could be so good with chickpeas starring as the main ingredient! Side note: This makes excellent cookie dough.

1½ cups cooked organic chickpeas
½ cup natural peanut butter
⅓ cup maple syrup
2 teaspoons pure vanilla extract
½ teaspoon baking soda
Pinch sea salt
½ cup vegan chocolate chips

1. Preheat the oven to 350°F. Line a baking sheet with parchment paper.

2. In a high-powered blender, blend the chickpeas, peanut butter, maple syrup, vanilla extract, baking soda, and salt together until smooth, about 1 minute. Fold in the chocolate chips with a spatula or wooden spoon.

3. Roll the dough into equal-sized balls and place them on the prepared baking sheet.

4. Bake for 20 minutes, until golden brown. Enjoy!

COOKED PLANT-BASED RECIPE

avo-fudgsicles

PREP TIME: 8 MINUTES • TOTAL TIME: 8 MINUTES +12 HOURS • SERVES 6

This nutritious, dairy-free frozen dessert is a great way to get in some extra avocado—and all of the healthy fats they contain. As if you needed an excuse to eat more avocado!

1½ cups mashed ripe avocado (about 2 small avocados)
½ cup cacao powder
¾ cup plant milk
½ cup maple syrup
1 teaspoon pure vanilla extract
Pinch Himalayan salt
½ cup natural peanut butter

1. Place all the ingredients in a high-powered blender and blend until creamy.

2. Pour the mixture into ice pop molds and freeze overnight.

3. To remove from the molds, briefly run under hot water or wait a few minutes to unstick the sides.

NOTE: *If you're not using a high-powered blender, add a little extra plant milk to get to a smooth consistency.*

PREDOMINANTLY LIVING PLANT-BASED RECIPE

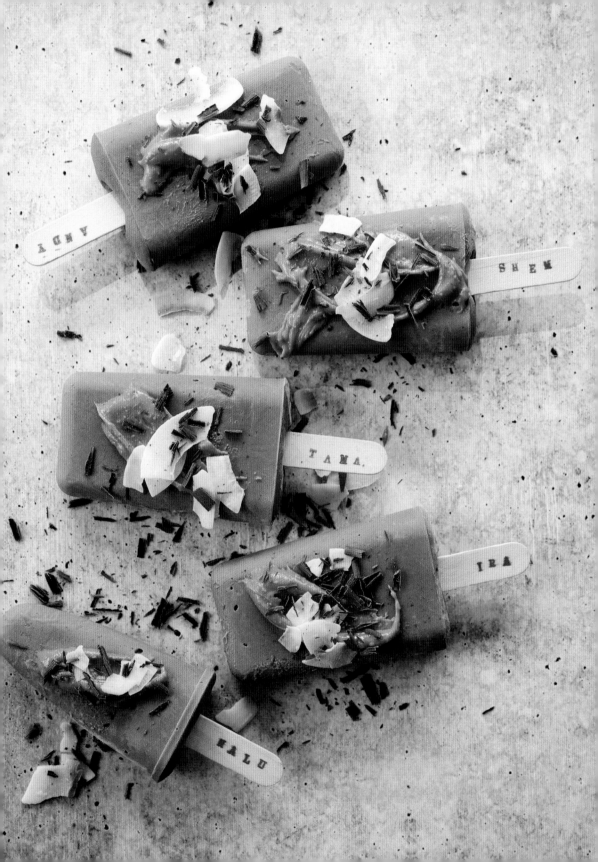

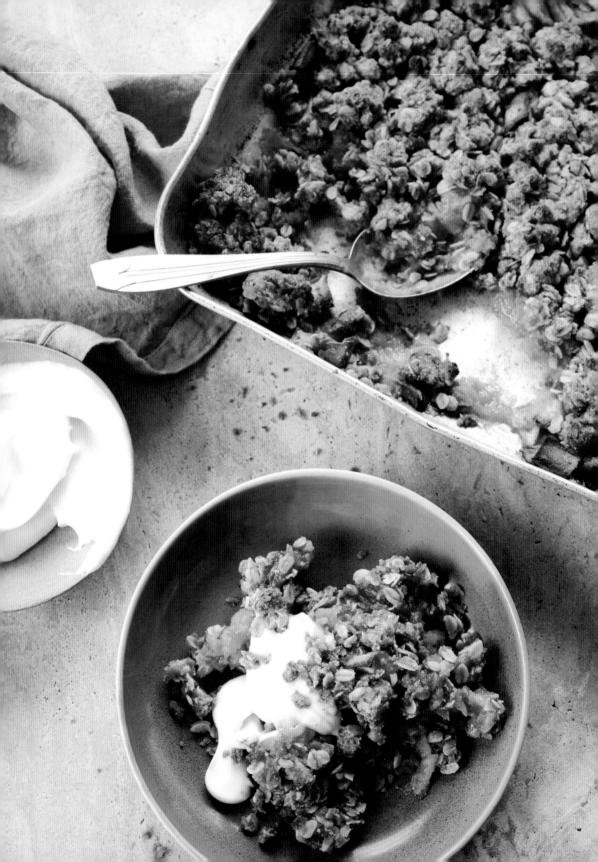

grandma's apple crisp gone vegan

PREP TIME: 20 MINUTES • TOTAL TIME: 1 HOUR 20 MINUTES • SERVES 8

This is my Canadian Irish mom's apple crisp recipe, plant-ified! Your taste buds won't know the difference, but your body will. Top with coconut yogurt or enjoy with a glass of cold oat milk.

¾ cup cold vegan butter, cut into small pieces, plus softened vegan butter for the pan
10 medium-sized Golden Delicious apples, peeled, cored, and sliced into ¾-inch pieces
2 cups old-fashioned gluten-free oats
1 cup all-purpose gluten-free flour
1 cup packed coconut sugar
1 teaspoon ground cinnamon
¼ teaspoon sea salt
Andy and Shem's Coconut Yogurt (page 92) for serving (optional)

1. Preheat the oven to 350°F. Lightly grease a 9 × 13-inch baking dish with the softened vegan butter.

2. Spread the sliced apples evenly across the bottom of the baking dish.

3. Combine the oats, flour, sugar, cinnamon, and salt in a large bowl. Stir the dry ingredients together, then mix in the chunks of cold butter, using your hands to create clusters.

4. Scatter the clusters loosely on top of the apples in the pan. Do not pack down (for the best texture).

5. Bake for 1 hour, or until the apples are soft and the top is golden brown and crisp.

6. Serve with coconut yogurt or enjoy as is.

COOKED PLANT-BASED RECIPE

hempies

PREP TIME: 14 MINUTES • TOTAL TIME: 50 MINUTES • SERVES 12

One afternoon my son Ira asked me if we could invent a recipe together. I said, "Of course!" and this recipe was born. Besides being drool-worthy and my all-time most popular recipe on social media, this easy treat requires no baking at all and just a handful of simple ingredients.

1½ cups plus 2 tablespoons smooth natural peanut butter
⅓ cup maple syrup or brown rice syrup
1 teaspoon pure vanilla extract
⅓ cup hemp hearts
3 cups organic crispy rice cereal
1½ cups vegan chocolate chips

1. In a large bowl, mix 1½ cups of the peanut butter, the maple syrup or brown rice syrup, and vanilla with a wooden spoon until smooth. Then stir in the hemp hearts and crispy rice cereal.
2. Line an 8-inch brownie pan with parchment paper and pat the mixture into the pan.
3. Combine the chocolate chips and remaining 2 tablespoons peanut butter in a medium microwave-safe bowl and microwave on high for 30 seconds, stir, microwave for an additional 30 seconds, and stir again. If it's not fully melted, microwave for another 30 seconds.
4. Spread the chocolate–peanut butter mixture evenly over the hemp and crispy rice base and put in the freezer to set for 30 minutes.
5. Remove, cut into 2-inch squares, and store in an airtight container in the freezer.

COOKED PLANT-BASED RECIPE

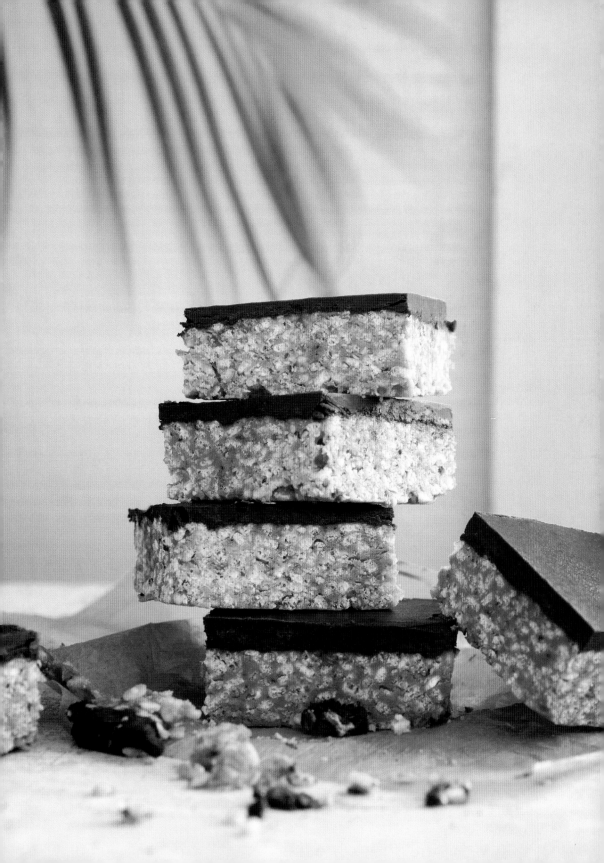

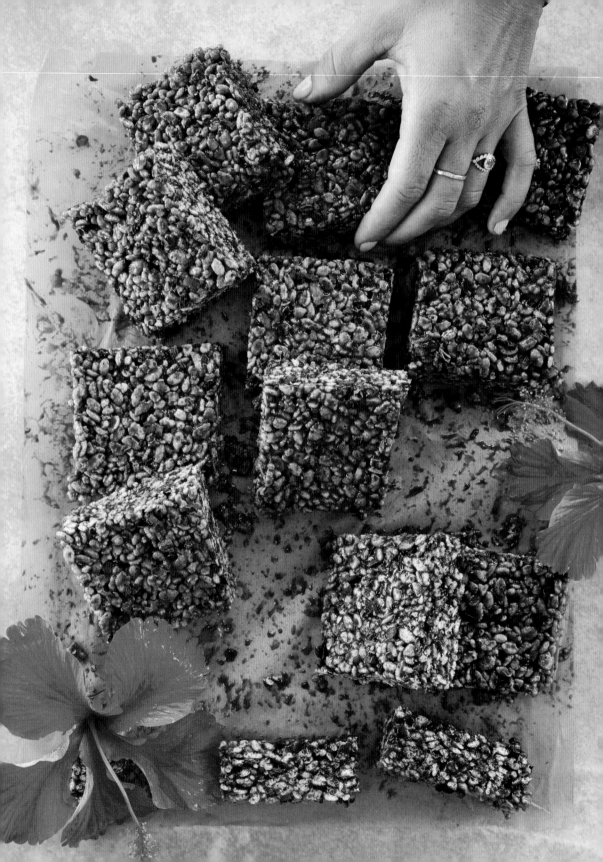

hippies

*Hippies are Hempies'
chewy chocolatey sister!
If you're a brownie lover,
you're going to flip over
this body-benefiting
alternative I learned from
Susan, a beautiful health
guru here on the North
Shore!*

1 cup maple syrup
1 cup brown rice syrup
1 cup your favorite natural nut butter
1 cup vegan dark chocolate chips
¼ cup coconut oil
9 cups organic crispy rice cereal
½ cup hemp hearts
¼ cup cacao nibs
½ teaspoon Himalayan salt

1. In a medium saucepan, combine the maple syrup, rice syrup, nut butter, chocolate chips, and coconut oil. Heat over low heat for 5 minutes, stirring constantly, until everything is melted and combined.

2. In a large bowl, combine the crispy rice cereal, hemp hearts, cacao nibs, and salt.

3. Gradually add the melted ingredients to the bowl with the dry ingredients and stir until well combined.

4. Grease a 9 × 11-inch brownie pan, pour in the mixture, and evenly spread it over the pan. Gently press until the mixture is firmly packed.

5. Place in the fridge to set and cool for 1 hour.

6. Cut into 2-inch squares and store in an airtight container in the fridge for up to 2 weeks.

COOKED PLANT-BASED RECIPE

raw chocolate mousse cake

PREP TIME: 20 MINUTES • TOTAL TIME: 20 MINUTES + 6 TO 12 HOURS • SERVES 12

A recent summer when we were in the Mentawai Islands, we had this insane raw vegan chocolate mousse cake, courtesy of my dear friend Chef João, who is making the world better with his drool-worthy vegan foods. Naturally, I had to learn the recipe for myself and share it with you!

FOR THE BASE:

2 cups unsalted almonds or peanuts
2 cups pitted Medjool dates
¼ cup cacao powder
½ teaspoon sea salt
2 tablespoons cacao nibs
1 tablespoon coconut oil

FOR THE MOUSSE FILLING:

3 ripe bananas, sliced
¾ cup packed coconut sugar
⅓ cup cacao powder
3 tablespoons coconut oil
1 (14-ounce) can coconut cream (not cream of coconut)

1. In a high-powered blender, blend the base ingredients on high until you achieve a chunky, paste-like consistency. It should be sticky. If it's too dry, add a bit more coconut oil.

2. Line a 10-inch springform pan with parchment paper and press the base paste into the pan.

3. For the mousse filling, blend the mousse filling ingredients in a high-powered blender until very smooth, like whipped cream.

4. Pour on top of the base.

5. Freeze for 6 to 12 hours. Slice and serve immediately. Or for a mousse-like texture, allow to sit at room temperature for 30 minutes before serving.

PREDOMINANTLY LIVING PLANT-BASED RECIPE

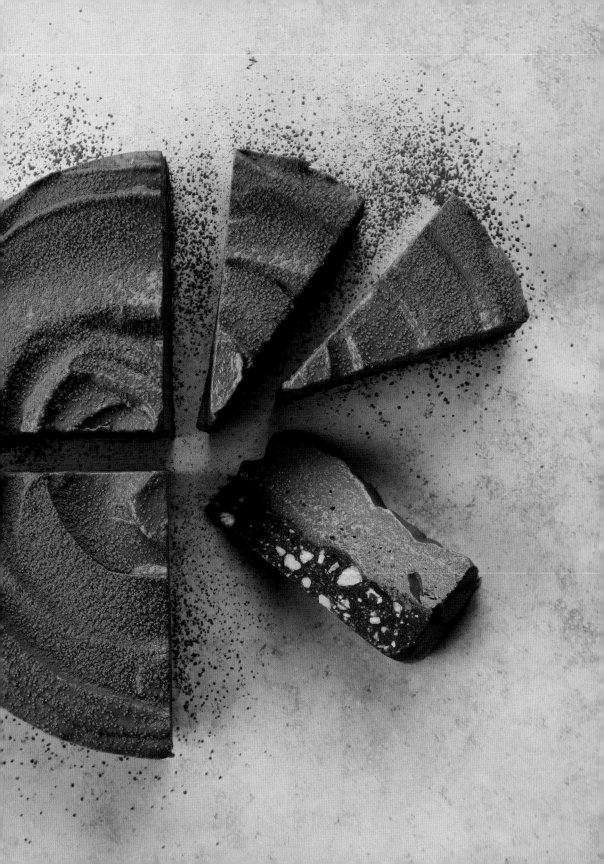

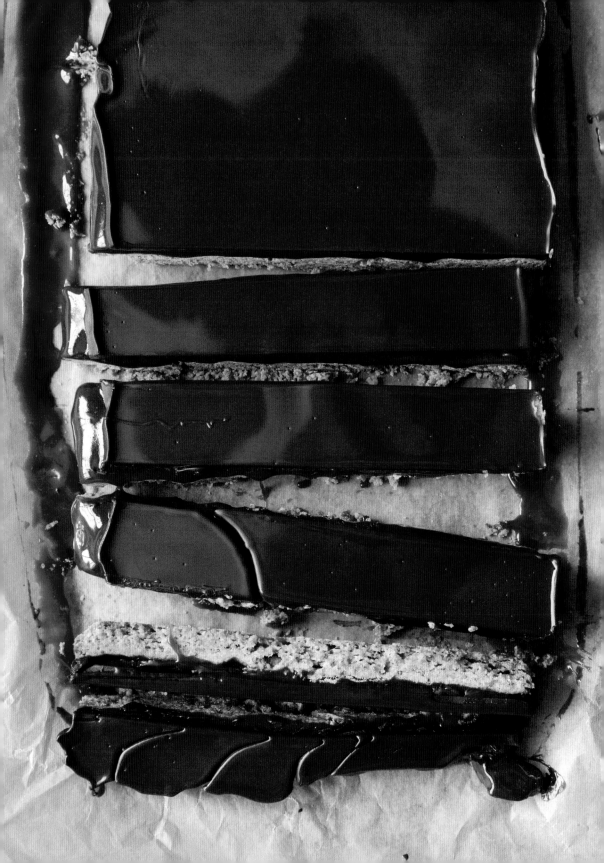

coconut caramel cookie bars

PREP TIME: 20 MINUTES • TOTAL TIME: 20 MINUTES + 2 HOURS • SERVES 14

Think gooey salted caramel center with a crunchy, light cookie crust, covered in coconut cream chocolate. Is your mouth watering yet? And yes, part of the process is licking the bowl of caramel clean.

FOR THE BARS:
2 cups all-purpose gluten-free flour
1 cup packed coconut sugar
½ teaspoon baking powder
1 teaspoon sea salt
1 cup coconut oil, melted and cooled

FOR THE TOPPING:
2 cups coconut sugar
2 cups coconut cream (not cream of coconut)
½ teaspoon sea salt
3 cups vegan chocolate chips

1. Preheat the oven to 335ºF.

2. To make the bars, combine the flour, coconut sugar, baking powder, and salt in a large bowl. Stir in the coconut oil.

3. Line a 9 × 11-inch baking pan with parchment paper. Press the mixture into the pan and bake for 25 minutes, or until crisp. Set aside to cool.

4. To make the topping, in a large saucepan, mix together the coconut sugar, coconut cream, and salt and heat over medium heat, stirring constantly until the mixture comes to a boil. Then lower the heat and simmer for 35 to 45 minutes, stirring constantly, until the sauce cooks down.

5. Test the consistency of the caramel by spooning a few drops from the saucepan into a cup of ice-cold water. If soft balls form when you pick up the drops between your fingers, the caramel is done.

COOKED PLANT-BASED RECIPE

6. Pour the caramel on top of the cooled bars. Set in the freezer to chill for 2 hours.

7. Microwave the chocolate chips in a microwave-safe bowl for 30 seconds, stir, then microwave for another 30 seconds to fully melt. Pour over the caramel layer, which will have set, and put back in the freezer to chill the chocolate layer for 30 minutes.

8. Cut into 2-inch squares. Store in an airtight container in the fridge for up to 2 weeks.

peggy's hawaiian chocolate chip coconut banana bread

PREP TIME: 25 MINUTES • TOTAL TIME: 1 HOUR 20 MINUTES • SERVES 10

My mother-in-law, Peggy, is a banana bread genius, and she has lovingly baked hundreds of loaves of her famous banana bread over the years for family and friends. She was kind enough to create this delicious gluten-free vegan version for me and to share it with us for this book. Thanks, Peggy!

FOR THE BANANA BREAD:
¼ cup plant milk
1 teaspoon apple cider vinegar or white wine vinegar
1 cup gluten-free all-purpose flour, plus more for the pan
½ cup packed coconut sugar
1 teaspoon aluminum-free baking soda
½ teaspoon sea salt
1 cup mashed overripe bananas (2 to 3 large bananas)
½ cup vegan butter, softened
2 vegan egg replacers (see Note)
1 teaspoon pure vanilla extract
1 cup vegan chocolate chips
½ cup unsweetened coconut chips

FOR THE GLAZE:
1 cup powdered sugar
1 tablespoon almond milk, plus more if needed

NOTE: *I like Bob's Red Mill Egg Replacer best as an egg substitute. If you can't find it, you can make chia eggs (see recipe on page 231), but your bread will have a slightly denser consistency.*

1. Set an oven rack to the middle position and preheat the oven to 325°F.

2. In a cup or small bowl, combine the plant milk and vinegar. Stir well and set aside for 10 minutes.

3. In a large bowl, combine 1 cup of the flour, the coconut sugar, baking soda, and salt.

4. In a separate bowl, combine the mashed bananas, vegan butter, egg replacer, and vanilla.

5. Add the wet ingredients to the dry mixture and stir to combine well.

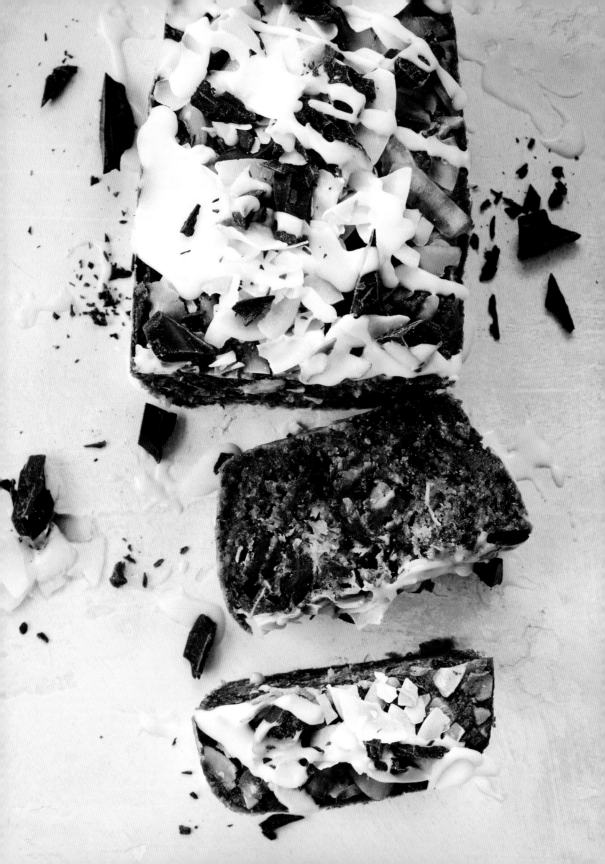

6. Lightly flour an 8½ × 4½-inch loaf pan. Pour in the batter and sprinkle two thirds of the chocolate chips and two thirds of the coconut chips over it. Take a fork and lightly mix the chocolate chips and coconut into the batter. Sprinkle the remaining chocolate chips and coconut on top.

7. Place the pan in the oven and bake for 55 minutes. Test by inserting a skewer into the center of the bread loaf; if it comes out clean, the bread is done. Remove from the oven.

8. Cool the bread in the pan for 5 minutes, then turn the bread out from the pan to continue to cool on a wire rack.

9. To make the glaze, whisk the powdered sugar and 1 tablespoon of the almond milk in a small bowl to dissolve the sugar. Add a little more milk if necessary so the glaze is smooth enough to drizzle.

10. With a fork, drizzle the glaze back and forth across the loaf. Serve sliced warm or cold with a nice glass of oat milk. Store in an air-tight container for up to 1 week.

how to make a chia egg

PREP TIME: 2 MINUTES • TOTAL TIME: 7 MINUTES • MAKES ENOUGH TO REPLACE 1 EGG

This is a great vegan egg substitute for pancakes, waffles, quick breads, cakes, and more!

1 tablespoon chia seeds
2½ tablespoons filtered water

Put the chia seeds in a small dish and add the water. Stir and let rest for 5 minutes to thicken to a gel-like consistency.

COOKED PLANT-BASED RECIPE

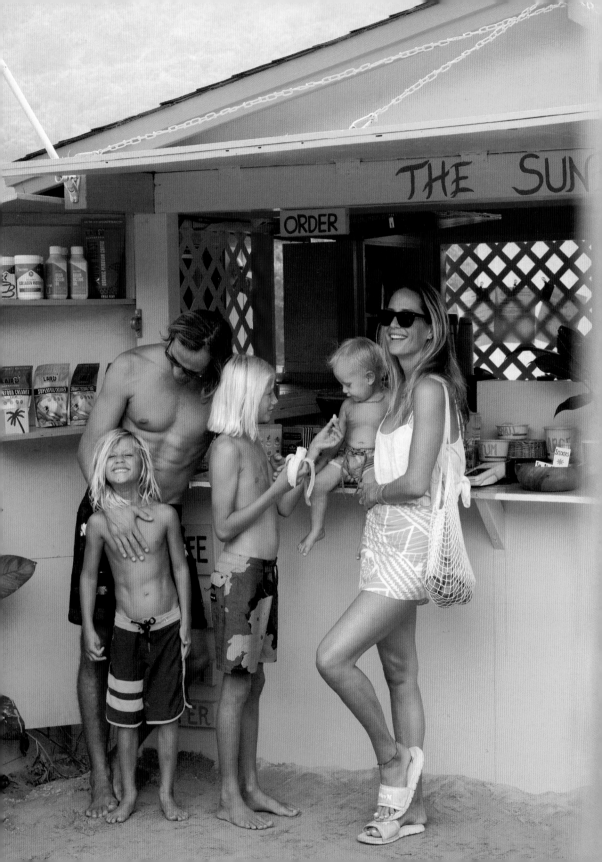

a whole new way of eating and living

Consistency is key to achieving long-lasting results, especially when it comes to our health. Adapting to a new, healthier way of eating takes time, but it will benefit all areas of your life—from the way that you feel about your body, to your energy levels, to your self-confidence and your relationships with other people. It's about changing much more than what you eat. It's about changing your entire mindset and your lifestyle. My life changed irreversibly when I made the connection between what I was eating and how I was feeling. I was thirty years old when I finally figured this out and began making the changes that were necessary to take back my health. I realized that my lifestyle choices could either support my health and my aspirations, or they could compete with them. I decided that I was going to live in a way that brings out the best version of me, and that allows me to be my absolute best for my family and the things that I care about most.

getting my family (and yours) on board

When I initially changed my diet four years ago, I did it by myself, for myself. But once I experienced the incredible physical benefits and realized that this was no longer an experiment but a way to live the rest of my life, I knew I had to get my family on board too. But that was easier said than done with a 6′ 4″ burger-loving husband and two (now three) young boys who are always hungry but who initially weren't thrilled about trading in their favorite snacks for fruits, veggies, and leafy greens.

The key to going Plant Over Processed, for yourself, and for your family, and making it work for you long term, is recognizing that change won't happen overnight. Perhaps surprisingly, it was harder to get Shem on board than it was to convince our boys! Picture me trying to get the boys to eat broccoli for dinner, and then Shem coming home from work and sitting down at the kitchen table with a tub of ice cream, or a bag of cookies! (This actually happened.) But eventually Shem came around, because he recognized how important these changes were to me, and he saw the benefits to our kids' health. And today he is as much of a believer in this way of eating as I am. If you have embraced plant-based and you are looking to get your whole family on board, you will need to be patient, and a bit sneaky. I started by purchasing fewer and fewer animal products and processed products at the market each week until, eventually,

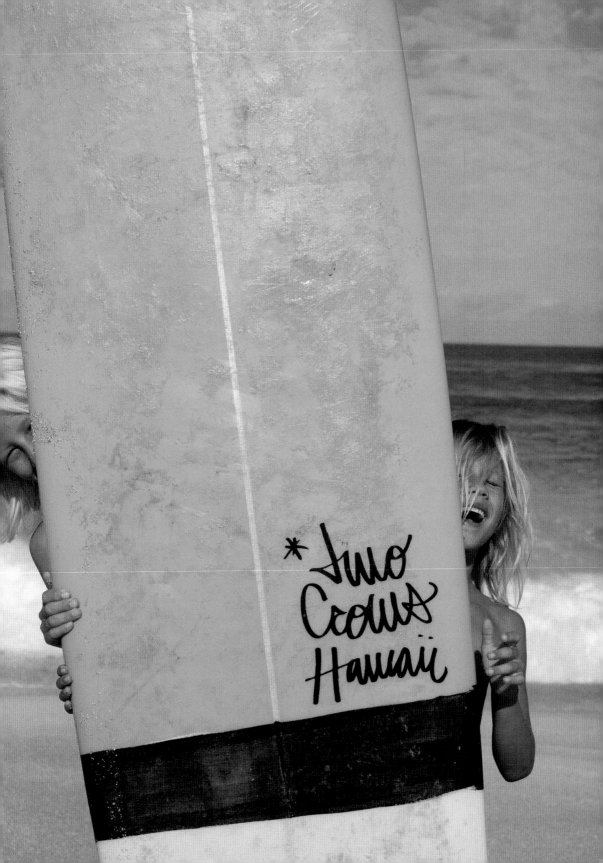

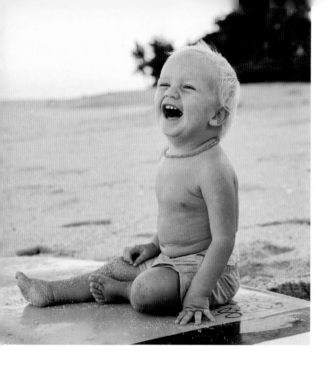

I wasn't bringing home any of these items at all.

You can do the same—gradually replace the items in your fridge and pantry, and start making plant-based swaps for your family's favorite meals slowly like I did: substitute coconut milk for cream; swap oat or almond milk for cow's milk; replace meat with vegetables in soups and stir-fries; use potatoes, avocados, rice, and beans in burritos and tacos instead of ground beef or fish. I made the cupboard and fridge health swaps over time. Each shopping trip, I'd swap out something like processed peanut butter containing high-fructose corn syrup for an organic natural peanut butter, refined sugar for coconut sugar and maple syrup, refined white flour for whole-grain or gluten-free flour, and so on.

Going plant-based had initially been about healing my own health issues, but after several months I saw the benefits for all of us. We were all getting sick less, the kids no longer had asthma or eczema, their energy and overall disposition improved, and Shem no longer had low energy, shaky hands, and chronic headaches. Today, particularly with the kids, I don't aim for perfection or being overly strict, but I do aim to have most of our calories come from plants. If my kids go to a birthday party and they are served cake with processed ingredients, they can decide if they want to eat it or not. My job and goal as a parent is to teach my kids to love healthy foods, and to understand where their food comes from. I want them to have a happy and healthy relationship with food and my hope is that they will continue to learn and make healthy sustainable choices for themselves for years to come.

Seeing the benefits of a plant-based lifestyle for my family has become my greatest motivation and it's my reason for sharing this journey. I'm a free spirit, and generally speaking I don't like a lot of rules! But there is one big rule in our house: Plant Over Processed. When we're hungry, we always aim to choose something plant-based (like a smoothie or trail mix) before we pick up something processed (like a cereal bar). I encourage you to do the same. Adopting this habit holds the potential to better your life!

why plant-based is better for mama earth

As I've mentioned, going plant-based was initially about doing what was best for my health, and for my family's health. But the more time that I spent living and eating this way, the more I began to think about the connection between our diet, our carbon footprint, sustainability, and eating ethically. I realized that every time I went to the grocery store, I was making conscious choices, voting with my wallet, and making decisions that would have an impact far beyond my own family and community. It was incredibly exciting to recognize how much more engaged and aware I had become! I never told my kids they couldn't eat animal products, but I did make it a priority to teach them about where their food was coming from, and I encouraged them to make healthy, plant-based, sustainable choices. It has been mind-blowing to see their interest in health, sustainability, and ethics develop. I am so proud!

Eating more consciously and sustainably is something that requires an open mind, and constant awareness of where our food is coming from. That may sound like a lot of extra work, but it is incredibly important, and it becomes a lot easier once you build healthy new habits. I think of eating consciously and

sustainably as a challenge that goes hand in hand with eating more plants. These decisions are connected, and I am always striving to be better! I encourage you to do the same.

Coming to terms with the way my food choices affect the planet has had very powerful consequences for me. Today, I often think about the fact that if my food choices were solely for health benefits, I might have fallen back into many of my old eating habits a long time ago. But recognizing the impact that our diets have on the environment

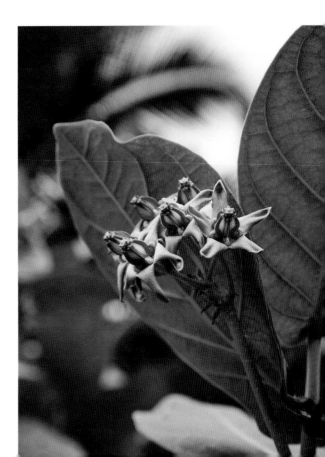

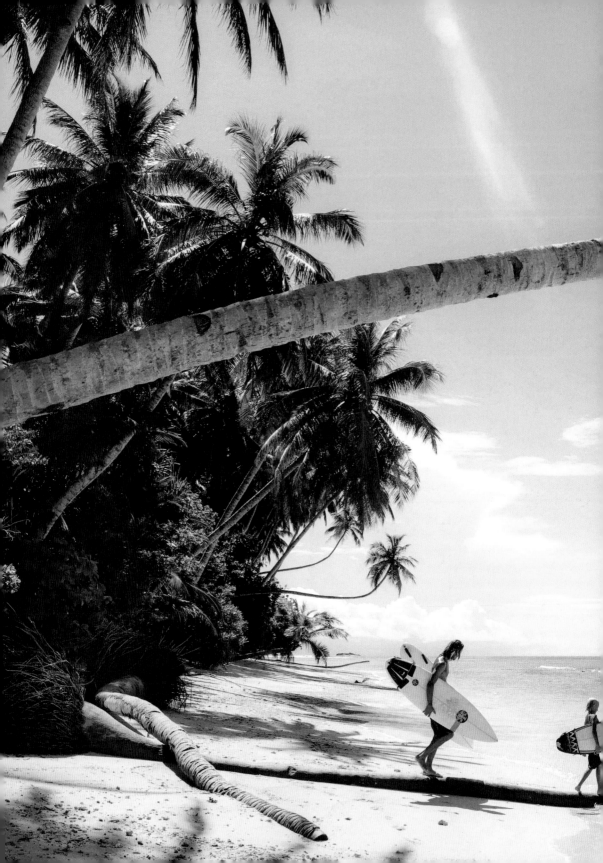

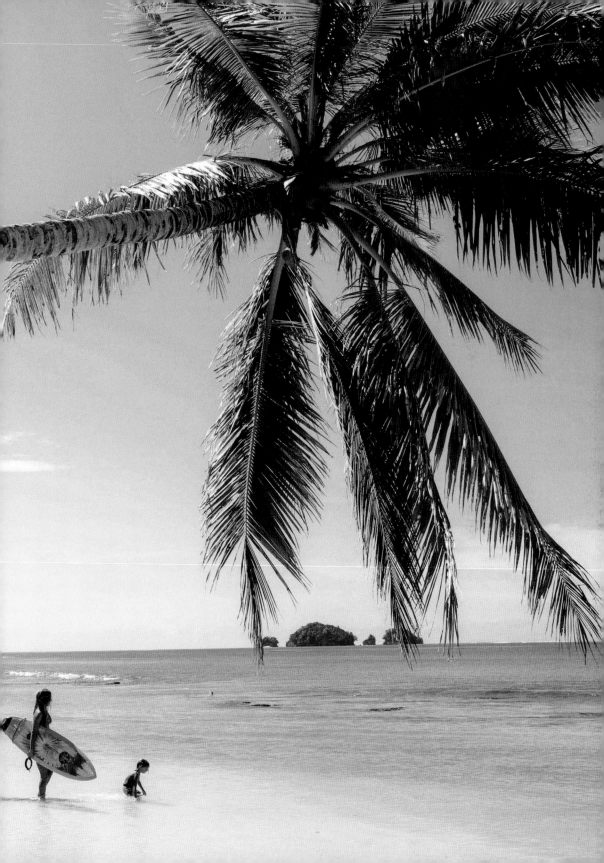

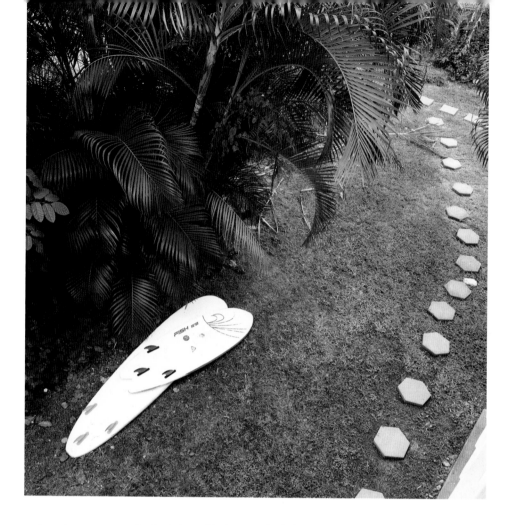

and on the treatment of animals has added an extra level of motivation for me. And many of the animal products that I once loved no longer hold appeal in the way they used to. I don't say this to make anyone feel uncomfortable or to pass judgment. As I've discussed, you may still choose to include animal products in your diet, and that is your choice. Our shared goal, at the end of the day, is to eat more plants!

I also recognize that being able to make the decision to eat a diet primarily made up of fresh fruits, vegetables, and other plant-based ingredients is a privileged one. Not all of us have the luxury of being able to make these kinds of lifestyle choices. Those of us who can make these conscious choices are incredibly fortunate—and all the more reason to express our gratitude for what we have been given by honoring this planet that we call home! With all of that said, let's take a look at some of the ways that going plant-based benefits Mama Earth.

the benefits of plant-based agriculture

It is well known that large-scale animal agriculture is a destructive force, and one that occupies over half of the world's arable land resources, using up an inordinate amount of our freshwater supply, and increasing greenhouse gas emissions that contribute to global warming. Additionally, the animal agriculture industry's pollution of the air, water, and land, coupled with land degradation and deforestation, causes a domino effect, leading to habitat loss for wild animals and pushing countless species to the brink of extinction.

Meat and dairy, particularly from cows, are the foods that contribute most significantly to global warming. Overall, beef and lamb have the biggest climate footprint per gram of protein, while plant-based foods have the smallest impact. Experts have concluded that a dietary shift toward plant foods and away from animal products is vital for promoting the health of our planet, not to mention individual human health. Studies have concluded that by giving up meat we can shrink our food-related carbon footprint by up to a third, and by giving up all animal products we reduce that even further.

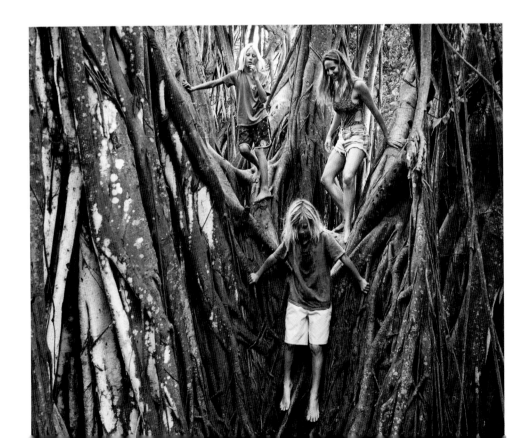

a plant-based diet saves water

If you are an earth-conscious individual you will find the Water Footprint Network enlightening. Check out their website (waterfootprint.org) for info on the impact that your lifestyle and dietary choices is having on the world's freshwater supply. For example, it takes approximately one thousand gallons of water to produce a single gallon of milk, and it takes one hundred times more water to produce a pound of animal protein than it takes to produce a pound of grain protein! If the world had an endless clean water supply this wouldn't be such an issue, but we don't.

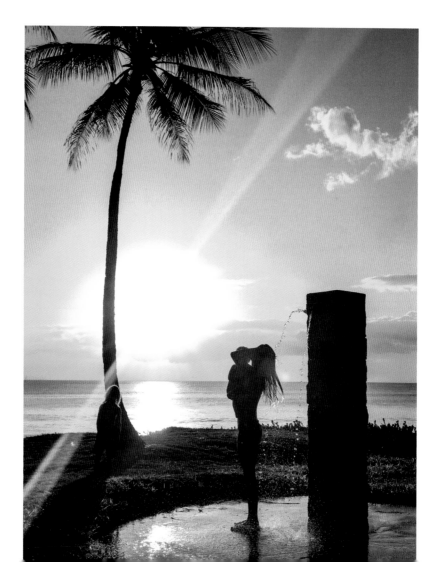

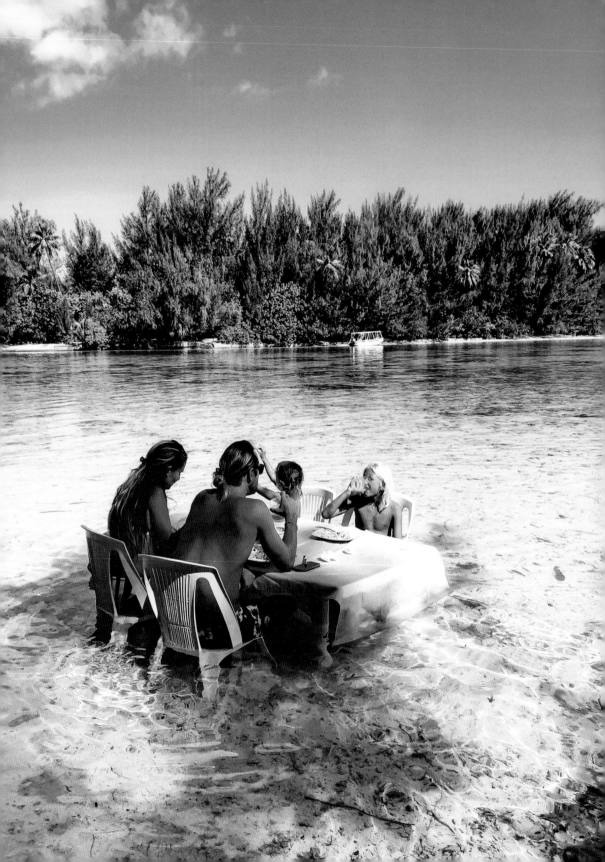

plant-based cuts down on plastics and packaging

The more natural, whole foods you buy, the less plastic packaging you bring home, and the less household waste you create. I was amazed at how much more time it took for our garbage bin to fill up after implementing a plant-based lifestyle. We used to empty our trash bin once every day. Now we'll go days before we need to empty it. I wasn't consciously trying to cut down on plastics when I began this journey—this was simply one of the added benefits of buying fewer processed foods and more produce. But as I became increasingly mindful of what I was buying at the grocery store, and the environmental impact of my choices, I challenged myself to find even more ways to reduce plastics and packaging in what I was buying and become more responsible about how I disposed of them. We have since learned to compost, save glass jars, and reuse what we can.

In 2017, my family and I took our first trip to the remote Mentawai Islands in Indonesia, and on this trip the negative impact of plastics and packaging on the environment really hit home for me. The natural beauty of the Mentawai Islands is astonishing, but while we were out surfing in the crystal-clear waters there, we'd see all kinds of plastic waste floating in the water. It was pretty upsetting! We also spent time in Bali shortly after our trip to the Mentawais, and we witnessed the same thing, only tenfold. After doing some investigation, I learned that what we were seeing was the result of the United States exporting boatloads of trash to Indonesia (as they do to other Asian countries as well) to be sold as raw and recycled materials. The trouble is, many of these materials are unusable, and they end up getting trashed again and making their way into the ocean.

Seeing firsthand how out of control plastic pollution has gotten in Indonesia really shifted my perspective. I came home from this trip committed to learning all I could about waste-free living and how we can properly dispose of the waste we do produce. Living in Hawaii, an island state surrounded by the ocean and so much incredible nature, has made me even more aware of the impact that my everyday choices have on the environment. In our local community, there is a fantastic organization called the Kokua Hawaii Foundation (KHF), founded by wife-and-husband team Kim and Jack Johnson, which runs a program called "Plastic Free Hawaii" aimed at minimizing single-use plastics on our islands. I am grateful to live in a community that supports environmental awareness, where even young children are learning how their habits can make a difference! But no matter where you live, you can become more aware.

YOUR LOW-WASTE, PLANT-BASED HOME

In order to eliminate unnecessary packaging and reduce waste, I've made some simple, everyday changes to my routine that I want to share with you! These are all so doable and easy; it's simply a matter of changing your habits (similar to the way we are changing our eating habits).

CREATE DESIGNATED RECYCLING BINS AT HOME. Place these right next to the garbage bin in your kitchen so that you will have no excuse for forgetting! Have a designated bin for recyclable glass, plastic, and aluminum, and a separate bin for paper and cardboard. The more conveniently located these bins are the better, so that recycling becomes a habit.

BYO GROCERY BAGS. Count the number of bags that you typically need for a single grocery haul, and make sure that you own and bring that number of reusable bags whenever you go to the store. I like mesh totes because they are so compact and incredibly easy to carry with you. I also strongly encourage you to bring your own cloth bags for bulk dry goods, and to bring jars for liquid bulk items. Grocery stores will allow you to

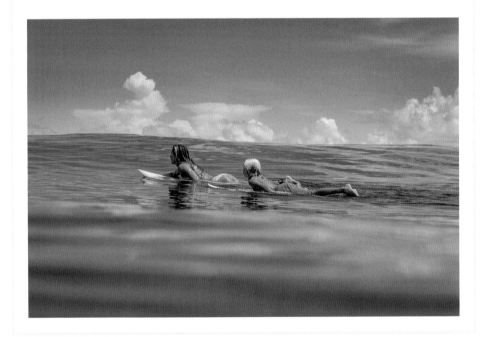

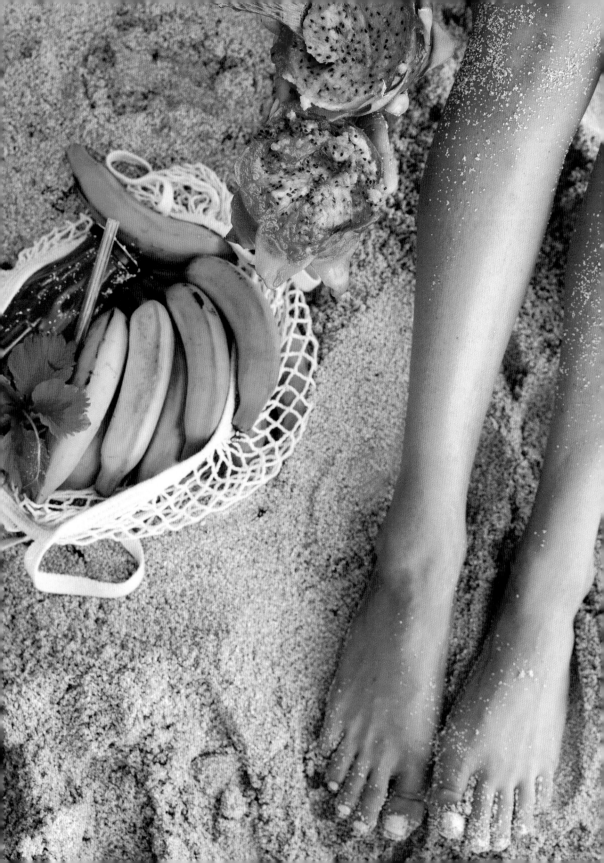

tare these storage vessels when you weigh your bulk items, and you will no longer go home with all of those single-use plastic bags—which end up in landfills, or in the ocean—after a trip to the grocery store.

SWAP DISPOSABLES FOR REUSABLES AT HOME. In your kitchen at home, swap those giant paper towel rolls for cloth kitchen towels, and replace paper napkins with reusable cloth napkins. Stop buying disposable plastic lunch and storage baggies and instead invest in a set of reusable silicone storage bags for snacks on the go. Use glass storage containers for snacks and leftovers at home.

USE DRINK BOTTLES. This one is obvious, but instead of drinking store-bought bottled water, or buying coffee, tea, and other beverages in single-use disposable cups or bottles, invest in a multipurpose, eco-friendly drink bottle that you can use for all beverages that you drink on the go. This is better for the earth, and it will save you money.

PACK YOUR LUNCH. For lunch on the go, instead of grabbing takeout or convenience foods, which inevitably come with packaging and waste, get a cool lunch box that you are excited about using with a set of reusable utensils and pack your own lunch! You will eat healthier, save money, and reduce waste—a triple whammy.

PLASTIC STRAWS . . . SUCK. As we now well know, plastic straws make their way into our waterways and are a danger to sea life. Many stores and restaurants offer paper or biodegradable straws, but this still creates waste! There's a simple solution: Buy a set of reusable stainless-steel straws online. There are even foldable options and straws that come with their own carrying cases for use on the go. I prefer stainless-steel reusable straws to bamboo and glass options, as they are easy to clean and won't break.

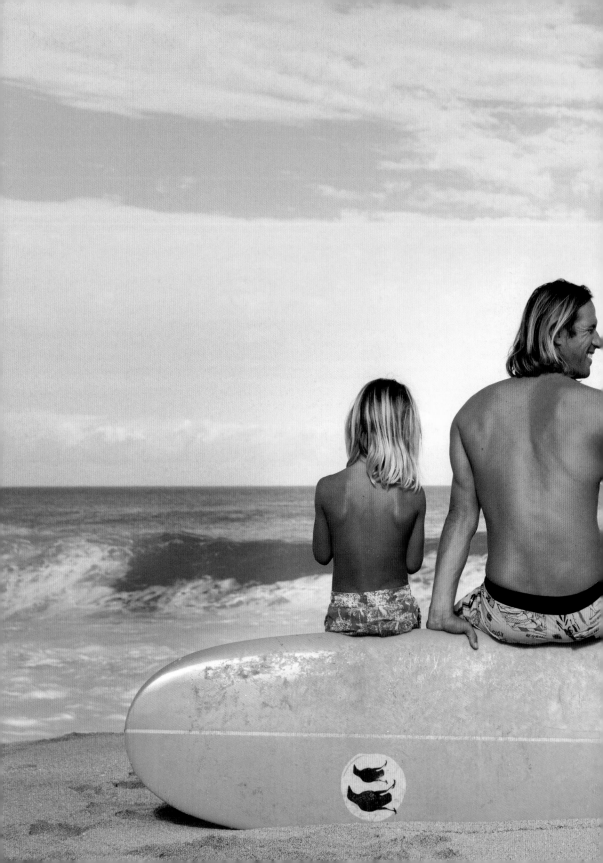

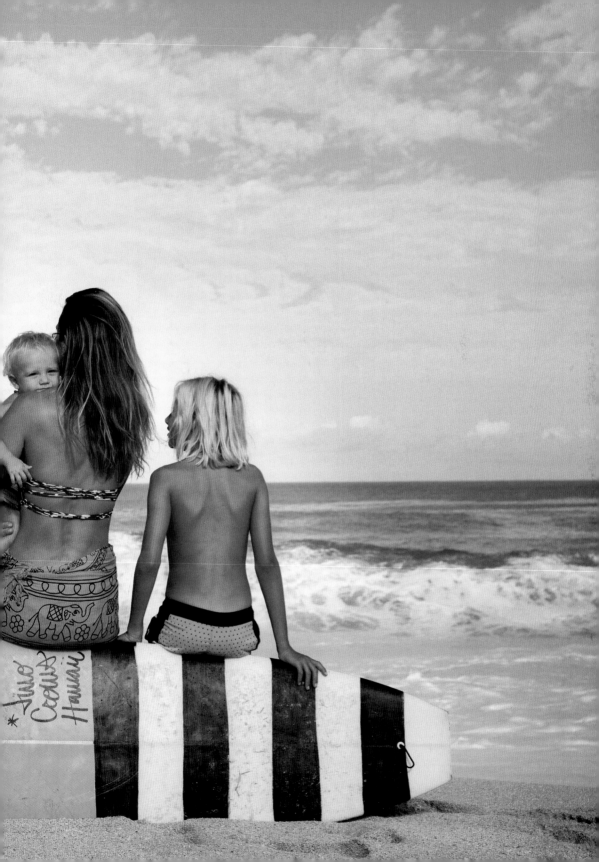

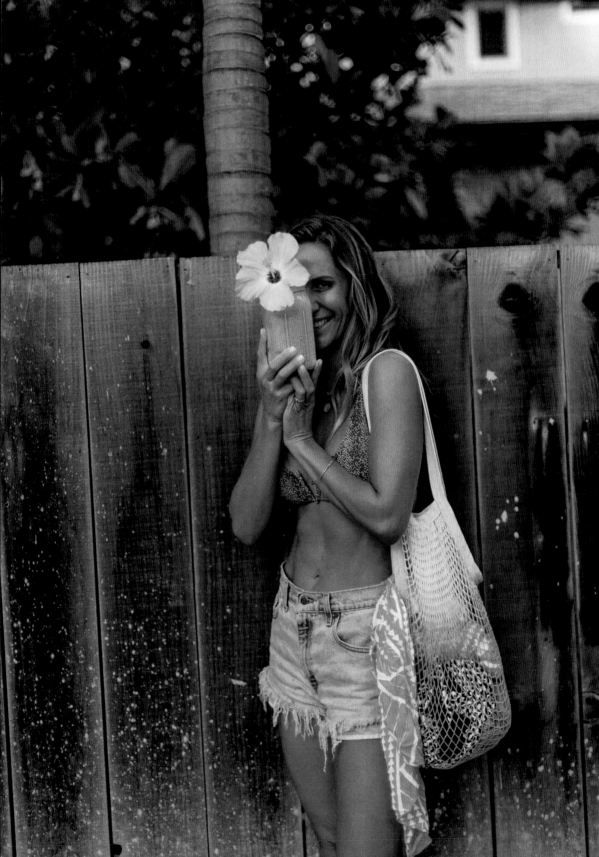

new
beginnings

Every morning we are born again.
What we do today is what matters most.
—BUDDHA

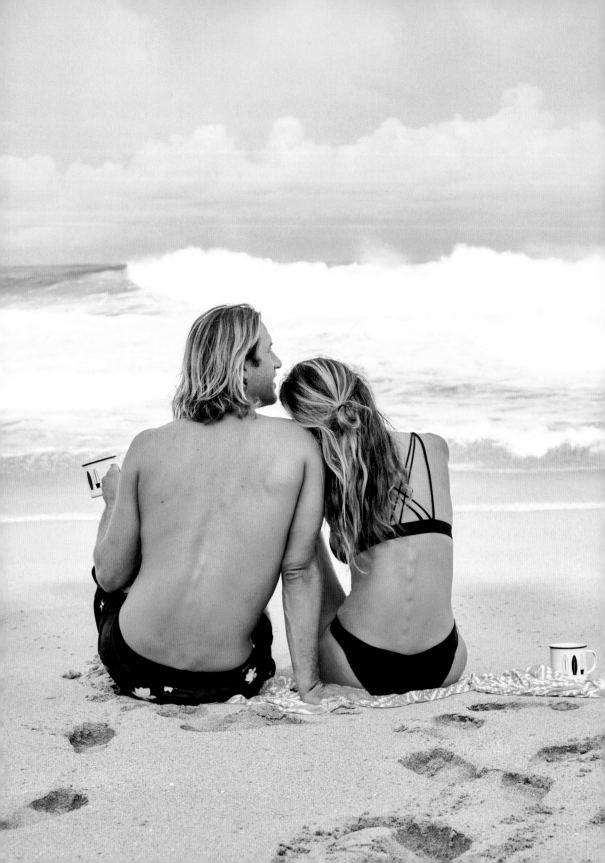

I hope that you have enjoyed this book's journey, and I hope that for you this is just the beginning! My aim has been to support and inspire you to embrace Plant Over Processed, and to help you learn to love living this way. Because this is about so much more than what you put in your mouth. It's about the connection between the foods you use to fuel your body, the way you feel, and your ability to live your best life as a result! We all know that if we don't feel well in our bodies, we can't show up and be our best for ourselves and for our families day in and day out.

The recipes in this book are meant to accompany you on this journey, to nourish your body and make you feel happy from the inside out—starting with your taste buds! I hope that my recipes, tips, and tricks will help you to get creative in the kitchen and that you will find favorite new dishes here to make time and again! I am genuinely excited for the changes that you are going to experience. The new sense of wellness that you will achieve with this way of eating is going to affect your life in all kinds of gratifying ways.

From this day forward, aim to eat more plants over processed foods, aim to make the connection with where your food comes from, and how that affects you and the planet you live on, and live in a way that reflects who you are and what you care about. Know that when you regularly consume wholesome foods, these foods will become your normal natural choice. All you need to do is eat them and they will do the rest. Plant foods will nourish you, take care of you, and can even reverse serious health complications. Over time your body will start to crave plant foods and thrive off of them. Consistency is the key to forming habits that will simultaneously change your lifestyle and your daily routines.

I know how hard it is to live without a sense of control over your own health. And I know firsthand how great it feels to make changes that put you back in the driver's seat when it comes to your health. Everyone deserves to feel good, and to eat nourishing, delicious, whole foods that heal and sustain the body. My wish for you is that you feel as great as I did after undertaking this journey. What may feel restrictive now is what will give you freedom later. I also want you to remember that Plant Over Processed is not about perfection. If you go off the rails, come back and restart! Ultimately this is about eating more plants, and fewer processed foods, whenever possible. You got this! Enjoy this process! It's a full-on adventure!

Sending you love,

Andy xo

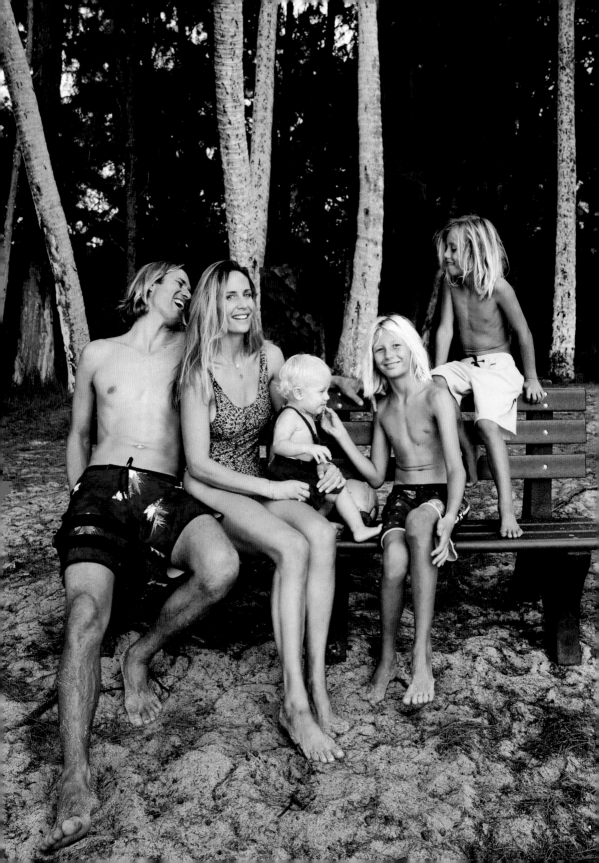

acknowledgments

To my family, my friends, and the Earthy Andy community, thank you for inspiring me every single day.

Thanks especially to my kids, Tama, Ira, and Nalu—you are the coolest and cutest little friends and taste testers I could ask for!

And to my husband, Shem, you are the acai to my bowl, but you already know that. Thank you for being my forever and my everything.

Thank you to my mom and my dad for teaching me how to work for what I want and to enjoy the process.

Thank you to everyone on my publishing team at Dey Street/HarperCollins. Special thanks to my editor, Jessica Sindler, and to my agents, Abigail Bergstrom and Megan Staunton, for your endless time, expertise, and encouragement. Writing this book has been a dream come true and I have you to thank.

Thank you to Petrina Tinslay for shooting the majority of the gorgeous photos in this book, and to David Morgan for styling all of the food so beautifully. You two truly brought the book to life! I had such a blast creating and spending memorable time with you.

Thank you, Amber Mozo, for all of the photos you have taken for me and my family over the years. I am so glad I could include them in this book. Thank you to Angie Prendergast-Sceats for helping me cook, to Logan Hollowell for adding sparkle to each picture with your jewelry, to Marie-Hélène Clauzon for your beautiful ceramics, and to Rose Daylight for creating the special utensils for my book!

Thank you to all my friends and family who taste tested, encouraged me, and inspired me, and who continue to be lights in my life!

Thank you to my managers, Kirstin and Rebecca, for always being there for me and my family and for keeping me sane.

And a giant thank-you to my readers. I am so incredibly grateful to you, and I hope that you find health and joy in this book!

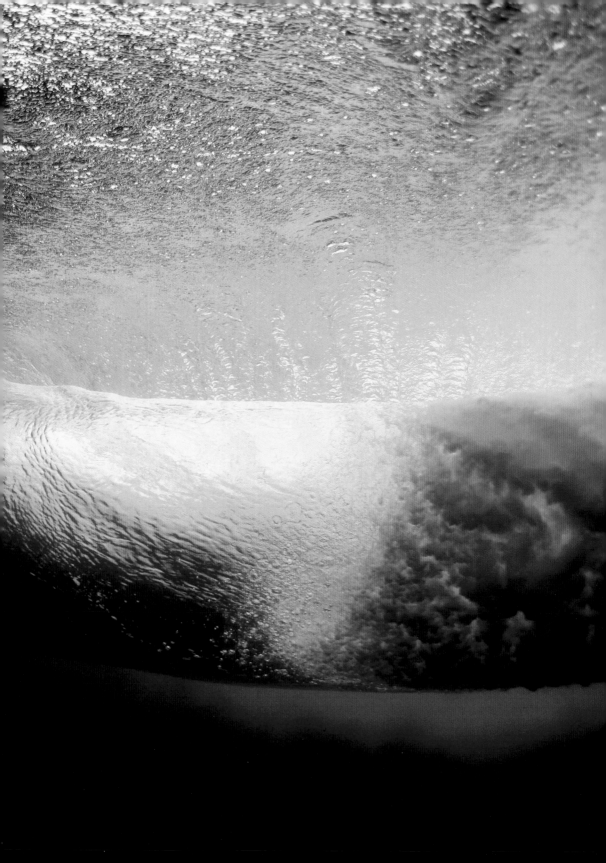

index

NOTE: Page references in *italics* indicate photographs.

C

DEY ST.

Photo credits: Pages iii, vii, 21, 28, 59, 123, 142–143, 233, 238–239, 250, and 256: Amber Mozo; vi, viii, 8, 16, 22, 32, 81, 83, 214, 242, and 243: Shem Hannemann; 61: Tahei Roy; 245: Damea Dorsey; 5: Tama Hannemann

All other photos by Petrina Tinslay

This book contains advice and information relating to health care. It should be used to supplement rather than replace the advice of your doctor or another trained health professional. If you know or suspect you have a health problem, it is recommended that you seek your physician's advice before embarking on any medical program or treatment. All efforts have been made to assure the accuracy of the information contained in this book as of the date of publication. This publisher and the author disclaim liability for any medical outcomes that may occur as a result of applying the methods suggested in this book.

PLANT OVER PROCESSED. Copyright © 2020 by Andrea Hannemann. All rights reserved. Printed in the United States of America. No part of this book may be used or reproduced in any manner whatsoever without written permission except in the case of brief quotations embodied in critical articles and reviews. For information, address HarperCollins Publishers, 195 Broadway, New York, NY 10007.

HarperCollins books may be purchased for educational, business, or sales promotional use. For information, please email the Special Markets Department at SPsales@harpercollins.com.

FIRST EDITION

DESIGNED BY RENATA DE OLIVEIRA
FOOD STYLING BY DAVID MORGAN

Library of Congress Cataloging-in-Publication Data has been applied for.

ISBN 978-0-06-298651-1

21 22 23 24   LSC   10 9 8 7 6 5

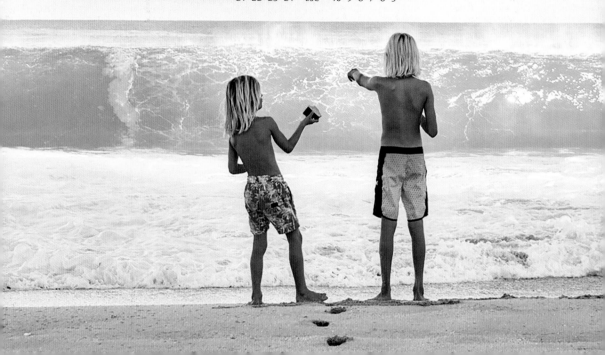